Kettlebell Training

Achieve Pain-Free Kettlebell T...
Foundation to Become a Professional Kettlebell Trainer

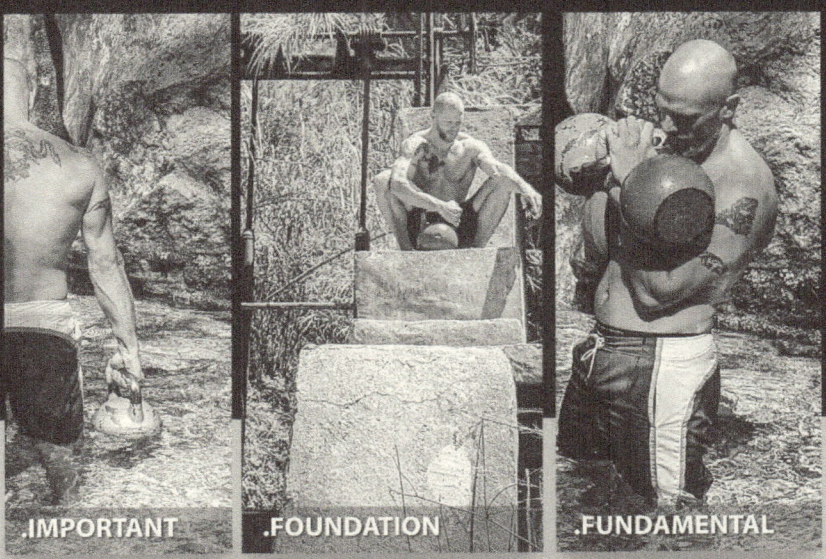

.IMPORTANT   .FOUNDATION   .FUNDAMENTAL

This is the first book in the series of kettlebell training by Cavemantraining, it covers fundamentals. Anyone not learning the fundamentals will run the risk of injury or giving up on training with the kettlebell.

You can pay a kettlebell trainer thousands of dollars and more than likely still will not learn all the finer details and little secrets that are explained in this book.

We've created a manual in which we explain how to reduce or completely avoid any aches and pains you might experience with exercises like for example; swings, cleans, lifts and presses. Learn how to avoid pain in the knees, elbows, wrists, shoulders, neck, lower-back, forearm etc.

This book is for people who experience pain or discomfort, it's to help reduce or eliminate callus, forearm pain and bruises, shoulder pain, elbow pain and much more when using kettlebells incorrectly.

An extremely good read. Recommended.
"A great addition to any kettlebell users library. I personally have gained more knowledge that will assist me with my journey using kettlebells as an enthusiast and an instructor."

Bryan Trish - kettlebell instructor and personal trainer

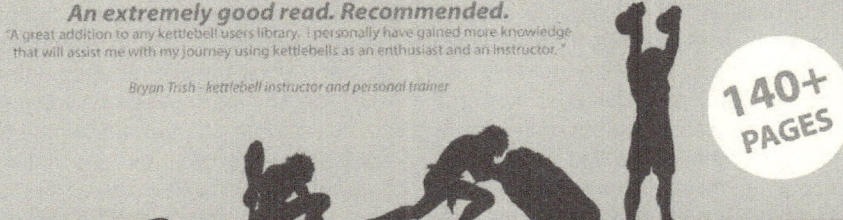

140+ PAGES

Written by the owner of Cavemantraining - Taco Fleur

KETTLEBELL TRAINING FUNDAMENTALS

Achieve Pain-Free Kettlebell Training and Build a Strong Foundation to Become a Professional Kettlebell Trainer or Enthusiast

This book is for beginners, trainers, or those who simply want to learn more.

Kettlebell Training Fundamentals is the first book in the Cavemantraining kettlebell series. Newcomers who fail to learn these fundamentals run the risk of injury, and unfortunately, may give up on kettlebells entirely.

Cavemantraining has published the following books and e-books in the Kettlebell Training series thus far:

1. Kettlebell Training Fundamentals (this book)
2. Kettlebell Grips & Racking (included in this book)
3. Racking (included in this book)
4. Master The Hip Hinge
5. Master The Basic Kettlebell Swing
6. Master The Kettlebell Press
7. Snatch and Swing Efficiency for CrossFitters
8. Kettlebell Workouts and Challenges 1.0
9. Flexibility, Mobility, and Strength Without Yoga

All books also available on iTunes, Amazon Kindle and in paperback format http://bit.ly/taco-fleur.

You could pay a kettlebell instructor thousands of dollars and more than likely still not learn all of the finer details and secrets explained here.

I will explain how to reduce or completely prevent any aches and pains you might experience performing exercises such as swings, cleans, lifts, and presses. Learn how to avoid pain in the knees, elbows, wrists, shoulders, neck, lower back, forearms, etc.

This book is for people who experience pain or discomfort from working with kettlebells; you can actually reduce or eliminate calluses, forearm pain and bruises, shoulder pain, elbow pain, and other maladies that result from using kettlebells incorrectly.

The most common exercises are covered in simple terms as well as intricate detail. You will not only find information on how to prevent pain, but why you need to do something a certain way will also be clarified; no one truly understands something fully until they appreciate the 'why' behind the explanation.

You will also find other details that you won't find elsewhere: for example, information about the many types of kettlebell grips available. It's hard to believe, but there are more than 25! And find not just a list of grips, but also an explanation for how to execute the grip and what they're most commonly used for. Any internet search will result in lots of information about grips, but it will also yield a lot of misinformation. I guarantee you that you won't find the solid descriptions based in practice and successful results that you will find in this book.

"A great book for anyone wanting to integrate kettlebells into their workouts. Taco covers a lot of information which will help you maximise your training. Links to videos are an added bonus and assist with the technical aspects of kettlebell training."

Mark Godwin
(Director, Fit Biz UK)

Valerie Pawlowski
World Champion Kettlebell Lifting

Master of Sport at Age 51 said:
"Well designed with good information. Nicely done"

An extremely good read. Recommended.

"A great addition to any kettlebell users library. Taco has done a great job with this easy to understand book covering many points on using a kettlebell with links to instructional videos too, very handy. There are very detailed descriptions on hand grips and racking a kettlebell as most books just cover exercises without covering the positions you and the bell need to be in. I personally have gained more knowledge that will assist me with my journey using kettlebells as an enthusiast and an instructor."

Bryan Trish
(Kettlebell instructor, Metafit Bootcamp, Circuit, Gym instructor and Personal Trainer)

"If you're a beginner, training in kettlebells or an instructor, it's definitely a go-to guide on how to start, if not perfect your journey into the world of KB sport.

Stumbling on to Taco's Facebook and connecting with him has turned my KB world upside down and made me even more excited about being in the industry - even after teaching KB for 4 years. This book is like having him in the studio with you. It's gutsy, honest and you won't walk away with 'but's and if's' because there are none. He says it like it is and you can either take it and advance yourself, or leave it and pretend like you know everything."

Lisa Colquhoun

About the Author

My name is Taco Fleur, and I'm an IKFF Certified Kettlebell Trainer, Kettlebell Level 1 + 2 Trainer, Kettlebell Science and Application, Kettlebell Sport Rank 2, CrossFit Level 1 Trainer, MMA Conditioning Level 1, MMA Fitness Level 1 + 2, Punchfit Trainer and Plyometrics Trainer Certified, with a purple belt in Brazilian Jiu Jitsu. I have owned and set-up 3 functional kettlebell gyms in Australia and Vietnam, and lived in the Netherlands, Australia, Vietnam and Thailand. I'm currently living in Spain.

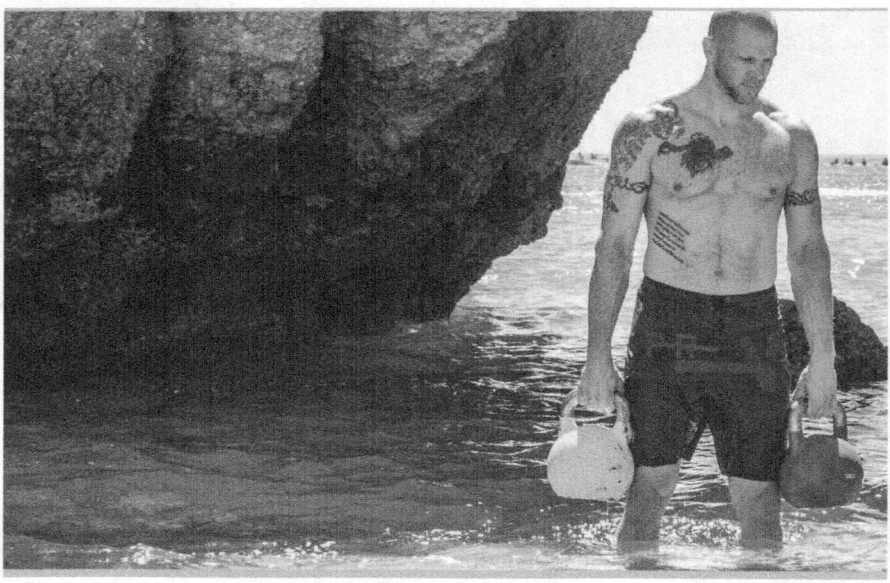

The first thing I'd like you to know about me is that I do not know everything, I don't pretend to know everything, and I never will. I'm on a path of life-long learning. I believe there is always something to learn from someone, no matter who they are. I've been physically active since the day I arrived on this earth in 1973. I got serious about training in 1999, touched a kettlebell for the first time in 2004, and got serious about kettlebell training in 2009. I'm here to do what I love most, and that is to share my knowledge with the world.

Some of my personal bests are 400 burpees performed within one hour; 500 kettlebell snatches, 500 swings and 500 double-unders completed in one session; 250 alternating dead clean and presses in one session with 20kg; 200 pull-ups in one session; 200 unbroken kettlebell swings with a 28kg; most kettlebell swings completed in one session with a 28kg (1,501); most total kettlebell swings done in 28 days with a 28kg (11,111); windmill with a 40kg kettlebell; lugged a kettlebell up a 1,184m mountain; 160kg dead lift; 250 alternating dead clean and presses in one session with 20kg; 100 snatches on sand with a 24kg kettlebell, 85kg Olympic Squat Snatch. I mention these PBs not to boast but to demonstrate that I have a good understanding of technique and movement across different areas.

My own training and goals are geared around GPP (General Physical Preparedness) which involves kettlebell training, calisthenics and CrossFit. I like high-volume reps but also like greasing the groove now and again. My main goals are to remains as agile as possible, remaining mobile, training in as many planes of movements as possible, and learning as many different exercise combinations and movements as possible while having fun and enjoying Brazilian Jiu Jitsu. I'm no Arnold Schwarzenegger and never will be, but strength is not solely defined by physical appearance and huge bulging muscles.

You can read more about my training, philosophy, and other ramblings on my website,

WWW.CAVEMANTRAINING.COM,

and on my YouTube channel, bit.ly/youtube-cavemantraining, which as of this writing has over 20,000 subscribers and more than 4.5 million views.

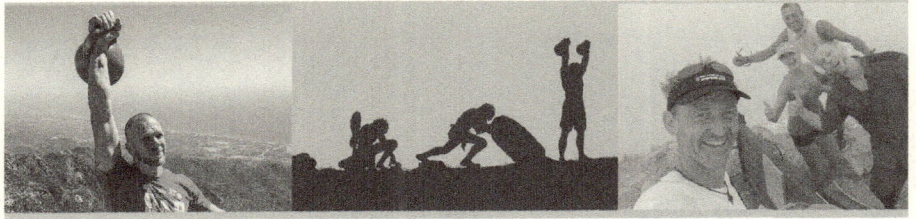

Add me: *Facebook.com/taco.fleur*
or Facebook.com/coach.taco.fleur
Facebook.com/Cavemantraining
or Facebook.com/Cavemantraining.
Magazine **for up-to-date articles and news.**

Please note that this material may not be reproduced or publicised elsewhere without the written consent of the author me@tacofleur.com.

If you bought this as a PDF/electronic copy, it is digitally signed and password protected with identifiable information.

All Cavemantraining owned images are copyrighted © Cavemantraining

> *Note: Most of the kettlebell stock images used in this book have literally been created with blood, sweat, and tears - I'm talking lugging kettlebells for hours up mountains, through canyons, running out of water, etc. Please respect the effort that has gone into producing the photos.*

Photos are available for purchase or in some cases made available for educational purposes with appropriate credits/links in return.

My writing style, explained. I believe it's important to describe the style of writing I employ. I like to keep things basic, covering the most important points using plain language and providing explanations where that's not possible. I like to repeat certain points in different contexts, as I believe this assists with retention of important information.

Subjects related will be put together in sections which I like to separate with a decorative line break, like so:

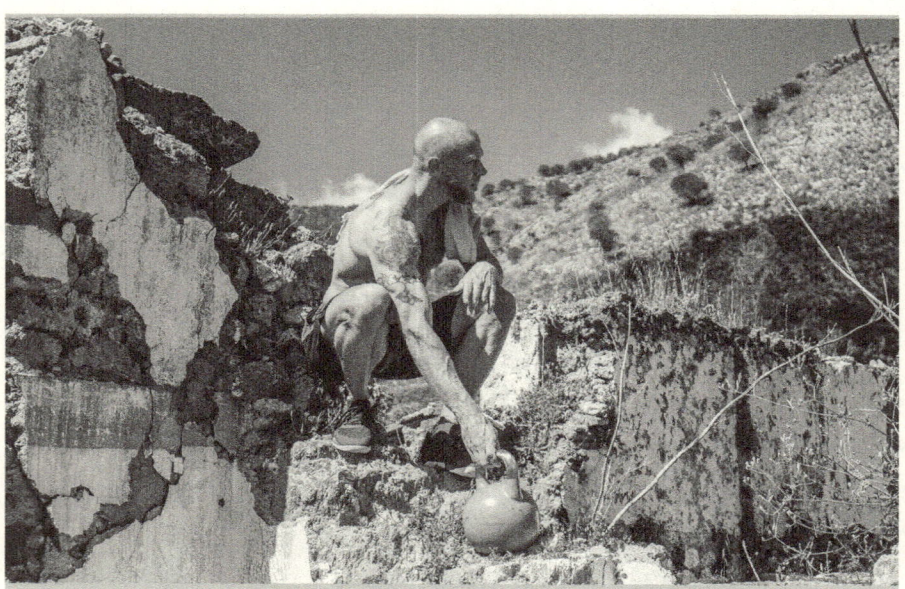

If you have any questions in relation to this book please do not hesitate to post those on our Facebook page or the Kettlebell Enthusiasts discussion group.

/caveman.training

/kettlebell.enthusiasts

Biased

I love kettlebells! If I was on a mountain carrying a kettlebell and a friend required carrying down, I would carry both down, and leave no kettlebell (or man) behind! That's a bit of an exaggeration... I would probably come back the next day to pick up the kettlebell, but I have heard people say that it looks like my kettlebells are like a member of my family, and they're not wrong.

You might wonder why I am bringing this up. If I was reading a book about a subject I cared about, I would want to make sure the author was not biased (i.e., writing only what he thinks is best). I started out with training in the gym many years ago. I used machines, bodyweight, and many other techniques and equipment, but once I started using kettlebells, I chose to make them my specialty, because I see the results they bring and the versatility they offer. In other words, I promote and love kettlebells, because I have experienced that for most people they are the best path to fitness.

If you think that means kettlebell training is all I want to do and all I will teach, you're wrong. I continue to educate myself and train in other disciplines as well, like CrossFit and anything else that inspires me. What I write is not based on dogmatic thinking, but years of research, experience, and results.

Feedback

I'm extremely open to constructive feedback, and I hope you will take a few moments to submit yours via email at education@cavemantraining.com or directly at me@tacofleur.com.

Review

If this book delivered what it promised, I hope you'll take a few moments of your time to leave a good review on Amazon, Cavemantraining, or Facebook. I would seriously appreciate it, it also allows me to see who is reading my book and what they truly think.

I truly hope that this book will provide you with information,

tips, and tricks to train with kettlebells safely,

and the ability to teach others.

So, without further ado...

Table of Contents

Kettlebell Training Fundamentals 2
  What is Kettlebell Training? 11
    Kettlebell Training Benefits 13
    Are Kettlebells Effective? 17
    Why Train? 18
    Working out Versus Training 21
  Kettlebell Safety 22
    Are Kettlebells Safe? 26
    Avoid Getting Hurt 26
    Progression is Key 27
    Progression for Beginners. 28
    Are Kettlebells Bad for Your Shoulders? 29
    Are Kettlebells Bad for Your Back? 29
  Warming Up for Kettlebell Training. 31
    Why Warm-Up? 32
    Focus. 32
    Mimic the Workout. 33
    Why Increase the Temperature? 33
    Why Increase the Blood Flow? 33
    Duration. 34
    Increase of Intensity and Complexity 34
  Which Kettlebell to Choose and Why? 36
    What Weight to Choose? 38
  Kettlebell Grips 40
    General Grip Information 41
    Why Should You Learn about Grips? 41
    Why Use Different Grips? 42
    Anatomy of the Kettlebell 43
    Hand Position on the Handle 44
    45 Degree Angle 45
    Grip Categories 47
    Double Hand Grip 48
    Swan Grip. 49
    OK Grip (AKA 2 or 3 Finger Grip) 50
    Corkscrew Grip 51
    Closed Double Hand Grip 53
    Hook Grip (AKA Overhand Grip). 54
    Closed Hook Grip (AKA C grip) 55
    Why Use Hook Grip? 55
    Racking Grip 57
    Racking Safety Grip 58
    Flat Hand Grip 59
    Pinch Grip 60
    Farmer Grip 61
    Bottoms Up Grip. 62
    Horn Grip 63

  Horn Grip Upside Down 64
  Corner Grip 66
  Open Hand Horn Grip 67
  Loose Grip 68
  Interlocking Grip 69
  Stacking Grip. 70
  Open Palm Grip 71
  Waiters Grip 72
  Goblet Grip.. 74
  Crush Grip 76
  Thumb Grip (AKA Noob Grip) 77
  Thumb Up or Thumb Down? Performance Gain? 78
Basic Double Arm Swing Instructions 82
  Squat and Hip Hinge Definition 88
  Swing Squat vs Hip Hinge Style 91
  American vs Russian Swing. 95
  The Problem with the American Swing. 95
Kettlebell Racking and Cleaning 99
  Why Rack Properly? 99
  Common Grips in Racking 100
  Kettlebell Clean 101
  Assisted Clean 101
  Swing Clean 106
  Dead Clean 111
  One Bell Racking Position. 111
  Bodyweight Racking Practise 112
  Spine Position for Racking 112
  Racking Points and Cues 114
  Kettlebell Resting Position 114
  The Racking Concept. 115
  Racking Types and Racking for Females. 116
Kettlebell Pain 119
  Muscle Aches 119
  Calluses 119
  Forearm Pain and Bruises 120
  Shoulder Pain 124
  Wrist Pain. 124
  Knee Pain. 124
  Elbow Pain 124
  Neck Pain. 126
  Lower-Back Pain 126
Kettlebell Golden Rules 127
Overhead Press. 130
Kettlebell Rows. 133
  Kettlebell Row Variations 134
  Muscles Worked with Rows 135
Stretching 136
  Butterfly Stretch 138

Lizard Pose ... 138
Tipover Tuck Hamstring Stretch ... 139
Easy Quad Stretch / Lying Side Quad Stretch ... 139
Kneeling Forearm / Bicep Stretch ... 140
Single Arm Chest Stretch ... 141
Posterior Shoulder Stretch ... 141
Overhead Tricep Stretch ... 142
Overhead Lat Stretch ... 142
Seated Leg Hug ... 143
Become Certified ... 144
Overseas Kettlebell Adventures ... 146

"Excellent document and the content is highly accurate."

~ Valerie Pawlowski
World Champion Kettlebell Lifting

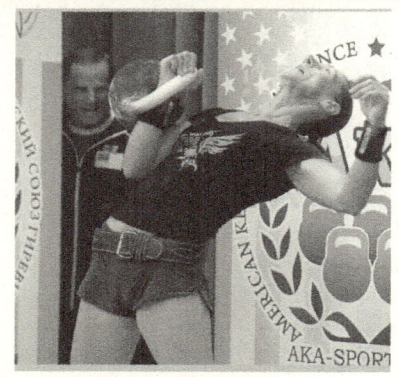

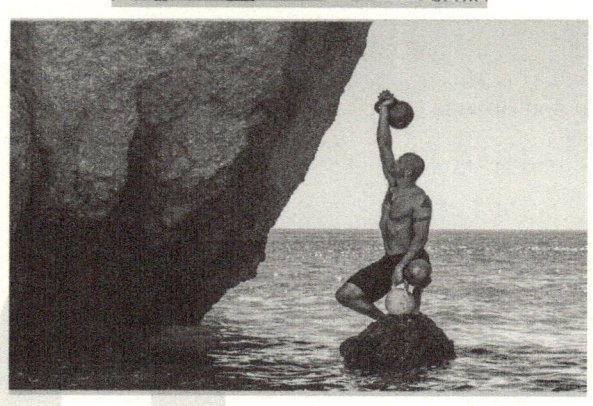

WHAT IS KETTLEBELL TRAINING?

A kettlebell is generally compared to a bowling ball (with a flat base) that has a handle. The weight of the kettlebell differs, but usually ranges from 8kg to 48kg in increments of 2 or 4 kg. Kettlebell training is a form of resistance training with the kettlebell providing the resistance. The goals that can be obtained with the kettlebell include, but are not limited to, cardiovascular fitness, flexibility, speed, power, strength, balance, mental toughness, etc.

Kettlebell training can get a bad rap due to the fact that many people just pick them up and fling them around, not realising that there is a precision and skill that should be developed step by step. Every exercise tool should be used with care and respect, and kettlebells are no exception. Kettlebells are extremely safe to work with, unless you use them recklessly, without instruction.

The kettlebell is truly a superior tool for workouts. I say this not just because I'm partial, but simply because it's a fact; there is no other tool as versatile that allows you train unilateral, ballistic, juggling and more.

If you're interested in the history of the kettlebell, you can view this video on our YouTube channel that I filmed with Steve Cotter while he was staying with me in Spain: https://www.youtube.com/watch?v=pDriaRWlLbs.

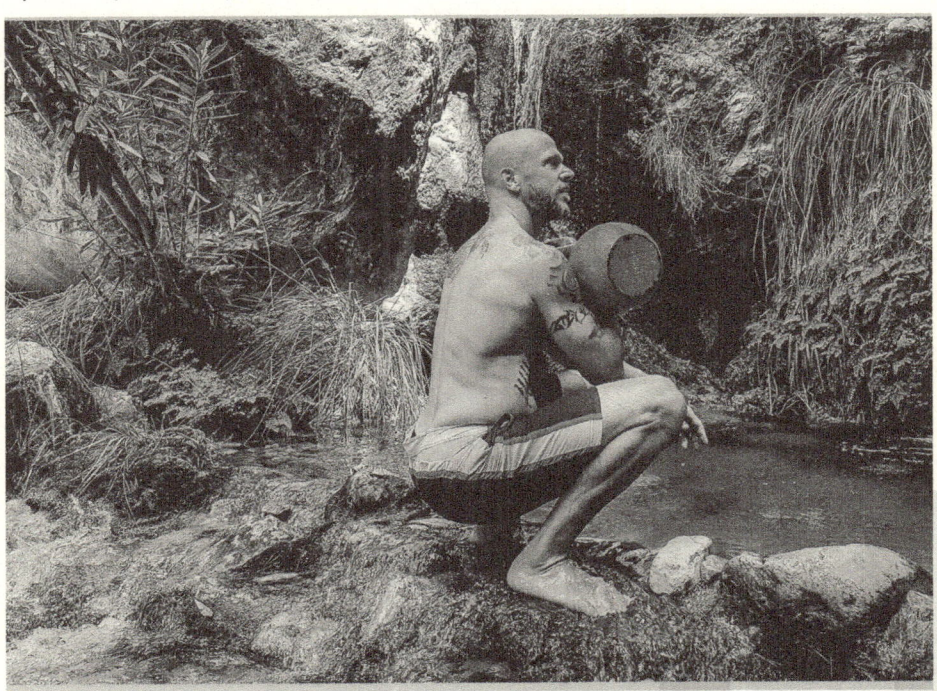

Taco Fleur in Rio Chillar, Nerja, Spain

There are several different organisations out there that all have their own methods of training; they all have their own style, and as far as I'm concerned, they're all good, if their teaching and intensions are genuine. In this book, I'm covering kettlebell training as *Caveman Kettlebells* which is Cavemantraining's best of all worlds . I'm mentioning all this to you, because you might find that some trainers will want you to do things a little differently; they might belong to RKC, StrongFirst, AKC, etc. I recommend that you keep an open mind, try it, understand it, use it; if it works for you keep it, if not, trash it.

I recommend that you not buy into just one organisation or train of thought - I don't subscribe to the "my way is the right way, and everyone else is wrong" philosophy. I like to train at other clubs, listen to other people, and learn as much as I can from everybody. I love kettlebells, and I firmly believe from experience that they're the best training tool you can find for all-around body conditioning, but I still use everything else at my disposal (including the barbell, which I believe is causing much more injury than any exercise tool out there at the moment, but that's for another chapter).

There are many who will disagree with my opinion, but the fact of the matter is, any type of training can cause injury when done incorrectly, and taught by people who don't know what they are doing. Take CrossFit for example: People get injured, but when it's done well, CrossFit can be an awesome and effective training regimen.

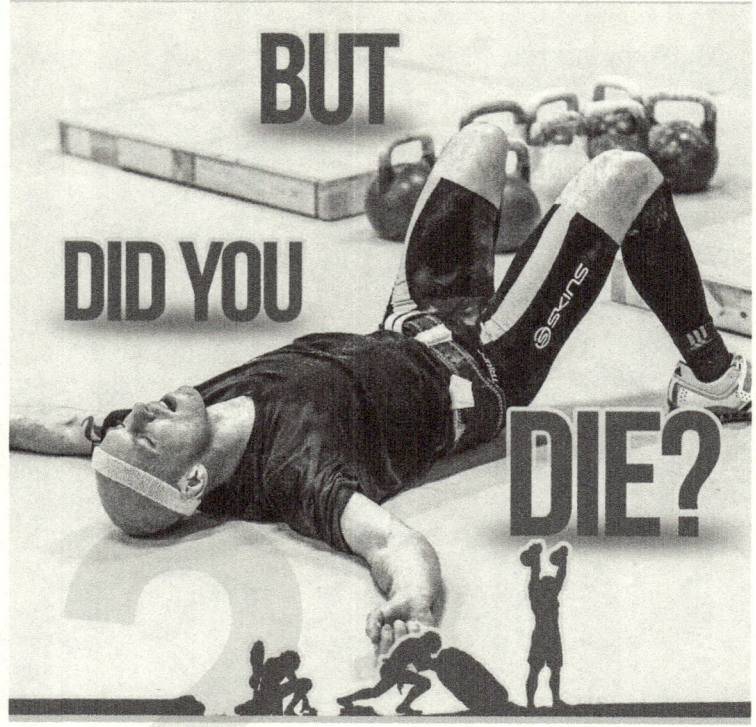

KETTLEBELL TRAINING BENEFITS

Why would someone want to train with kettlebells? To answer this question, one needs to know and understand the benefits provided through kettlebell training. Knowing the benefits will also help you sell your services if you become certified and choose to train other people; the benefits of kettlebell training combined with your professionalism and expertise will be the reason people will want to pay to train with you.

The following are some of the major benefits one will gain from kettlebell training:

- **Versatile**
One tool to work every muscle in the body
- **Complexes**
Due to the huge variety of kettlebell exercises available, the kettlebell is an awesome tool to create countless complexes
- **Portable**
Easy to carry and use anywhere
- **Compound exercises**
Work more than one muscle group with the majority of exercises
- **Unilateral**
Prevent muscle imbalance by working your muscles evenly
- **Cardiovascular endurance**
Gain strength while simultaneously improving your cardiovascular endurance
- **Functional**
Exercises that improve and assist in everyday movement
- **Flexibility**
Improve flexibility without the need to hold long and complicated stretches
- **Core muscles**
Improve strength due to constantly engaging core muscles during multi-plane movements
- **Fatloss**
Increase fat loss due to versatility of exercises, which provides increased calorie burn
- **Stabilizer muscles**
Works important stabilizer muscles normally neglected in training
- **Challenging**
Challenges both the muscles and the brain
  - **Fun**
  Never boring due to numerous exercises, complexes and workouts possible

- **Ability**

  Able to do more with newfound strength, power, flexibility, coordination, and endurance

- **Adaptable**
  - Everyone can work out with kettlebells, whether teenager or senior
  - Equally beneficial for men and women
  - Challenging for everyone from office worker to MMA fighter

- **Strong back**

  Helps prevent back pain and injury through improved engagement of posterior muscles not usually challenged

- **Multi-plane**

  Swing, press, pull, lift, and perform ballistic movements with just one tool

- **Time-Friendly**

  You can get a great workout in a relatively short period of time

Here is a bit more detail with regard to some of the aforementioned benefits:

Free Weights

Kettlebells fall under the category of "free weights" which include dumbbells, barbells, medicine balls, and sandbells. Unlike weight machines, they do not constrain users to specific, fixed movements, and therefore require more effort from the individual's stabilizer muscles. It is often argued that free weight exercises are superior for precisely this reason. For example, they are recommended for golf players, since golf is a unilateral exercise that can break body balances and requires exercises to keep the balance in muscles.

Compound Exercises

Kettlebells in general are used for compound exercises, it's not common to perform isolating exercises. Compound exercises mirror the ways that people naturally push, pull, and lift objects, and are therefore more functional and better for creating real strength in a person.

Unilateral

The most important aspect of unilateral training is the fact that it will help overcome strength imbalances. An example of a strength imbalance is pressing a 40kg Olympic barbell overhead with two arms, but the right arm is stronger and will push more of the weight. In other words, the right side might be pressing 25kg while the left is pressing 15kg. If you take one 20kg kettlebell and press it overhead with the right side, you will press exactly 20kg; if you press with the left it will be exactly 20kg.

A second example is a seated leg press: Two legs are pressing the 40kg weight at the same time, but the right side will probably dominate and press more weight than the left leg. If you now take a 20kg kettlebell and do a single-leg squat (pistol squat) with right and then left, both legs will have pressed the same weight. By using non-unilateral exercises, one can unwillingly produce muscle imbalances (i.e., the right side is usually more dominant and stronger, thus continuously pressing more weight than the left side). The dominant side continues to get stronger while the left gets weaker. Muscle imbalances makes a person prone to injury.

Unilateral exercises also challenge the core and stabilizing muscles more than bilateral exercises. Take, for example, one 20kg kettlebell (or other weight) in each hand and stand up. Stand there for a little bit, and focus on the feeling you get and what muscles you activate. Now, take only one 20kg kettlebell in one hand, and let it hang on the right side of your body. You should feel different muscles being engaged, in particular your obliques*, which are the muscles right above your hips and next to your abdomen. The obliques are engaged due to the unilateral aspect of the exercise; the weight will want to pull your torso (upper body) to one side, the side where the kettlebell hangs. Your body needs to engage the obliques on the other side to stop the torso from dropping to the side where the kettlebell hangs. If you train bilaterally (two weights), you will not get the same effect. This is just one example of a unilateral exercise, challenging only one muscle group, but there are many exercises and muscles challenged by unilateral training with kettlebells.

*Note that you have internal and external oblique muscles. Stabilizer muscles are not directly involved in lifting weight; instead they help keep your body steady when performing weight-resistance exercises.

Cardiovascular Fitness

Also commonly known as cardiovascular endurance exercises, or simply "cardio", which is the ability of the heart, blood cells, and lungs to supply oxygen-rich blood to working muscle tissue, and the ability of the muscles to use oxygen to produce energy for movement.

Non-Aerobic Exercise (also known as anaerobic exercise)

Exercise that is typically less than 60 seconds in duration, as opposed to aerobic exercise which is 60 seconds or longer in duration, like jogging 5 miles or going for a hike.

*Examples of aerobic exercises are running, cycling, rowing and many more.

The better a person's cardiovascular fitness is, the longer and more easily they can endure aerobic exercise. There are many kettlebell exercises, workouts, and complexes that can help improve cardio, but one kettlebell exercise in particular that seriously tests your cardiovascular endurance is the kettlebell swing.

Functional/Functional Training

Functional training attempts to adapt or develop exercises which allow individuals to perform the activities of daily life or sport more easily and without injuries.

Multi-Plane

Discussion of planes of motion can get quite complicated, but fortunately, in-depth knowledge is not required to understand this concept; a quick summary will suffice to get the point across.

Direction of movement can be split in three planes, sagittal, frontal, and transverse. Most forms of exercise do not take the equipment through all three planes and challenge the body from different angles. The kettlebell on the other hand, has exercises that travel through all planes and challenge the body from all different angles. The "snatch" is one great example of this versatility.

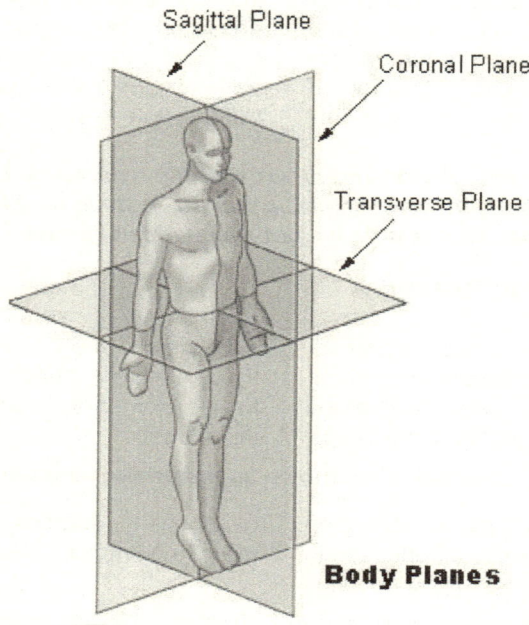

Body Planes

Strength Muscles vs Stabilizer Muscles

Kettlebell training works both the strength and stabilizer muscles, and produces an increased stabilizer muscle strength due to the multi-plane exercise possibilities, which in turn assists with greater overall strength unlike any other exercise equipment.

ARE KETTLEBELLS EFFECTIVE?

That's a great question, and one that newcomers should ask, but the answer is not simple. Whether they're effective or not depends on whether they can meet your goals, whether you put in the effort, and, most importantly, whether you use them correctly. Thus the final answer lies with you. Can they be effective? Without a doubt, yes!

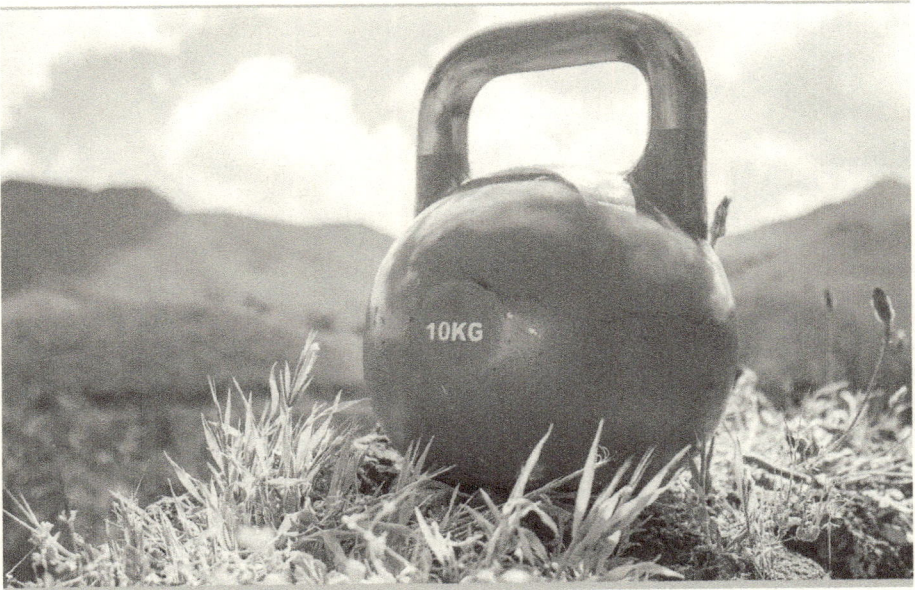

Training Basics

"There was a point in my life where I thought that knowing what muscle groups were worked and targeted in an exercise was futile; there was even a point where I thought that mirrors in the gym were just for posers. I did not have a great trainer to teach me otherwise. I had trainers who just rattled out how all the muscles worked but not explaining why, or perhaps not even knowing why, but just doing it because everyone else does it."

Taco Fleur

In the beginning of my career as a gym owner and fitness coach, I trained people that saw only part of an exercise pattern, the start and end phase, and thought that they were performing the pattern correctly as long as they got to that end phase in any way possible. I wish I had been better able to explain myself back then with more than just repetitive exercise correction.

I know now that in most cases understanding the WHY is more important than the correction itself. With this section I hope to get across to you the WHY for understanding muscles targeted, and the importance of using good form and technique.

WHY TRAIN?

✓ People train to develop and improve a physical ability through instruction from trainers and by practicing

✓ Each exercise is designed to produce a result, to target specific muscle groups and to put those muscles to the test

✓ Each exercise has a certain pattern, form, and technique that needs to be followed, or the exercise can become useless

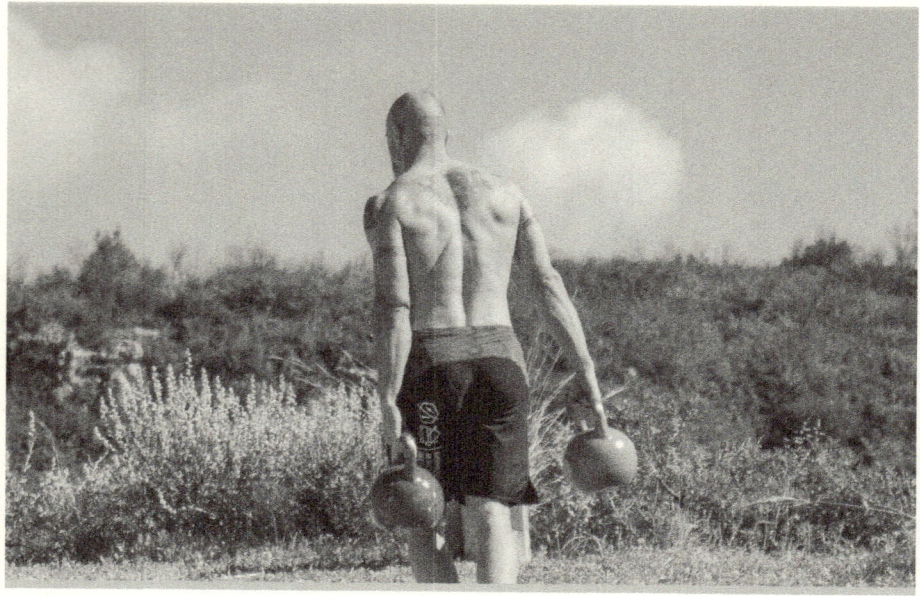

Let's take the squat as an example, as this is one of the exercises I have seen the most problems with. The primary muscle targets of the bodyweight squat are the quadriceps and gluteus maximus. The squat exercise is designed to improve leg strength and flexibility. In other words, the desired outcome of squatting is to be able to safely **squat heavier weight and go deeper**.

Proper form and technique is to pull yourself down into the squat while maintaining an upright torso; placing the weight on the quadriceps, the gluteus maximus is engaged to keep the pelvis upright, remove pressure from the spine and extend the hips. In the end phase of the squat, the hips should ultimately be past the knees when viewed side-on, the torso should be as upright as possible, the spine is neutral, the shoulders approximately aligned with the ankles, the knees in-line with the hips and feet. The up phase of the movement is powered by the quadriceps, hamstrings, and gluteus maximus.

Common Mistakes

Here is what I notice in many people. Without seeing themselves in a mirror and paying attention to the muscles they should be feeling, they end up in an end phase of the squat which looks like this:

- ✓ Torso leaning forward
- ✓ Shoulders past the feet
- ✓ Hips above or inline with knees
- ✓ Falling down into the squat
- ✓ Taking weight off the target muscles

The end result is a badly executed squat that puts more weight on the back muscles as opposed to the muscles targeted - the muscles that should have been worked in this exercise have almost totally been taken out of the equation.

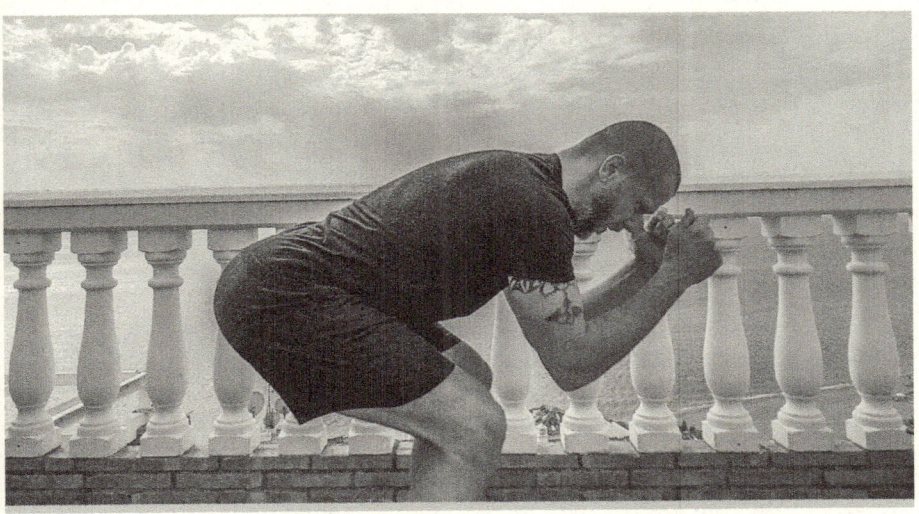

Badly executed squat, resembles more of a hip hinge movement.

In some cases people take a shortcut because they want to end up in the same position as the people next to them, or at least feel like they are, while they should be focusing on their own personal form and technique, building up strength and flexibility by only doing half the movement but keeping the muscles under as much load as possible. Each person needs to work at his/her own capacity in order to progress.

The point I'm making is not about the squat itself, but that one should **understand the goals** of an exercise, understand the form and technique required to execute the movement, understand the muscles targeted, understand the muscles powering the movement, understand the muscles assisting the movement, and ultimately understand the 'WHY' behind the exercise in order to progress to new levels of ability, which is why you're training, after all!

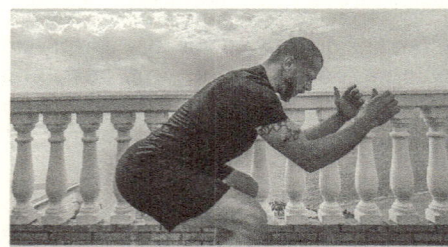 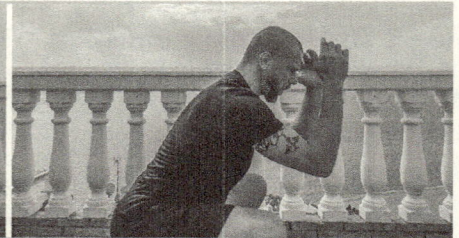

Improved. Better.

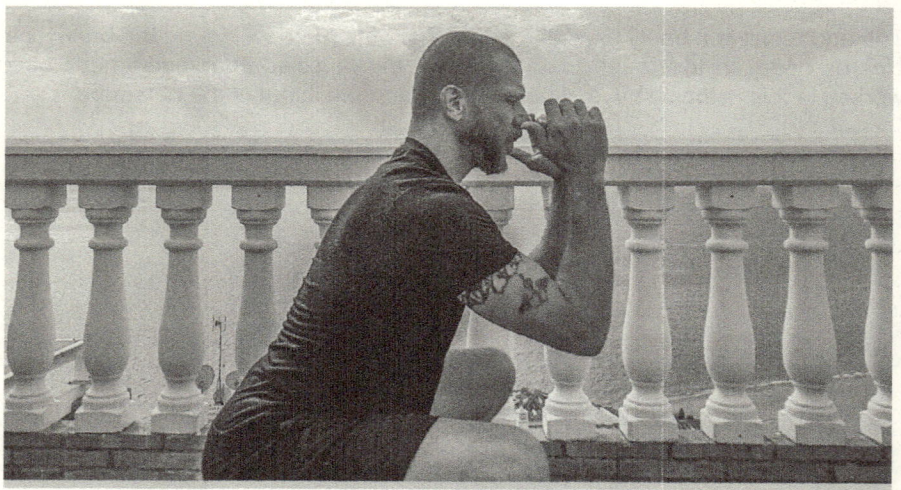

Best.

With that said, it should be noted that a lot of exercise movements can be powered using different muscle groups. This is not always a bad thing if it's intentional, works towards your goals, makes sense and is technically safe and sound.

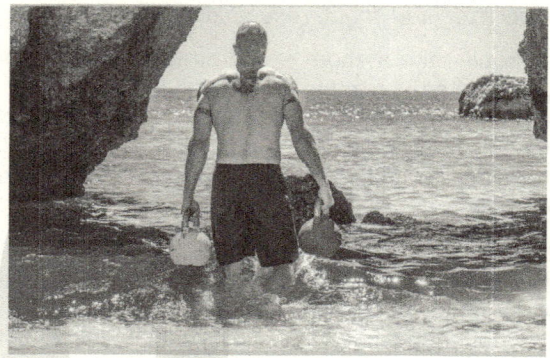

Taco Fleur in Lagos, Portugal

WORKING OUT VERSUS TRAINING

When you're training, you're getting specific. This means you're training a specific exercise or group of exercises—either under the guidance of a trainer or yourself—with the specific aim of improving. The goal of the training can be establishing better technique, getting more reps, or using more weight, but training is all about having a defined goal and a predetermined way to get there.

In contrast, when you're working out, you're performing a test of your general fitness. You're using the training you've undergone, and the aim is to "get your sweat on" while you find out what specific areas you might improve (i.e., train). In a workout, the focus is not about improving technique; it's about maintaining technique despite the grind and fatigue. The goals are to get a pump, feel exhausted, do more reps, beat a time, or compete against someone else.

In CrossFit, you could say the workout is the WOD, and the training, or those sessions done with your coach in private, is the EMOM. Because of the focus on improvement, training should always be performed slower than a workout; in training, every single rep should be scrutinized by your coach or yourself and the mirror—in a workout, you're going for it. So if you're exclusively participating in WODs, the fact is you're just **working out**, not **training** to get better. This means you're probably not making progress as quickly as you could, and might even be getting injured more frequently.

If this sounds like you, take a step back and ask yourself what your goals are. Trust me, it's time well spent—you'll never get to your destination until you know where you're going!

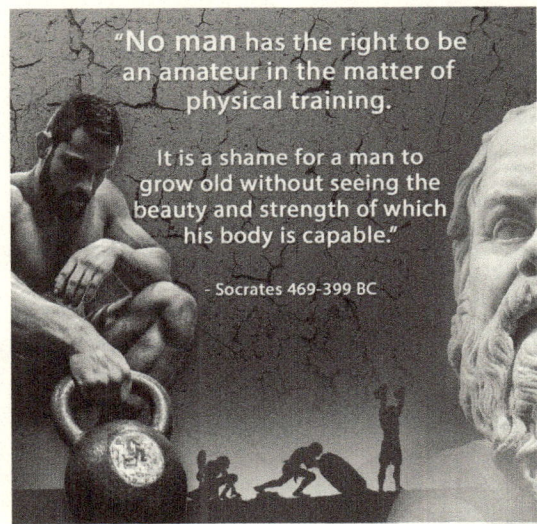

Eric Leija (left)

KETTLEBELL SAFETY

Be aware of your surroundings at all times; don't train too close to any mirrors, glass, walls, equipment, or other people. A 2-metre by 2-metre or larger area is preferred. Train on a flat, non-slip, dry area.

Communication is of the utmost importance. Communicate with your trainer or whomever you receive guidance from, and if something does not feel right, hurts, or is uncomfortable don't assume that the trainer can always see this. Express your issues; never feel shy or afraid to ask something; there are no stupid questions. If you're a trainer, it's important that you develop a rapport with your client and keep a close eye on him or her during each and every session. If the client appears to be having trouble, is in pain, or something is out of place, connect with your client and ask questions as simple as, "Are you ok?" in order to keep the lines of communication open.

Never try and rescue a bad repetition; you will only risk injuring yourself. If you lose control of the kettlebell when performing any exercise, don't try to rescue or catch it, but instead let it fall to the ground – the kettlebell will not break, and it's far better than being injured.

Some additional tips for keeping exercises safe and effective:

- Don't try to stop a swing in mid-air; instead let the swing finish
- Progress appropriately; do not rush progression, and regress when required (more on this later)
- Don't train to the point of complete exhaustion; rest when appropriate and before fatigue sets in
- Always protect your back by bracing your core on every rep
- Protect the shoulders by engaging your lats, and pull the shoulders down into the sockets
- Prevent hyper extending your back
- If it doesn't feel right, it's not right; stop what you're doing
- Maintain the calluses you develop on your hands
- Train in flat shoes or barefoot; running shoes do not provide stability during training and can cause injuries due to incorrect alignment
- Dry your hands when they get sweaty and/or use chalk
- Wear bandages/band-aids when you have cuts, not just for your own safety, but also that of others
- Listen to your coach or trainer at all times

Injury happens when you get lazy, fatigued, or don't listen to instructions.

Don't Get Lazy

When I mention laziness, I'm not referring to the fat slob type of laziness, so allow me to explain. When you perform a good swing, each rep requires effort; it requires activation of the glutes, hamstrings, lats, lower trapezius, middle trapezius, rhomboids, and much more. When you get lazy and don't put in effort, you will be using the minimum number of muscles to make the movement – this is the type of laziness I'm referring to. You have the strength to use the required muscles, but you choose not to because it's easier.

On the flip side, when there is actual fatigue, meaning you know what muscles to engage but you're simply not able to due to exhaustion, this is not the same laziness. Either can get you injured. Don't get lazy, and if you are so tired you can't perform an exercise correctly, take a break.

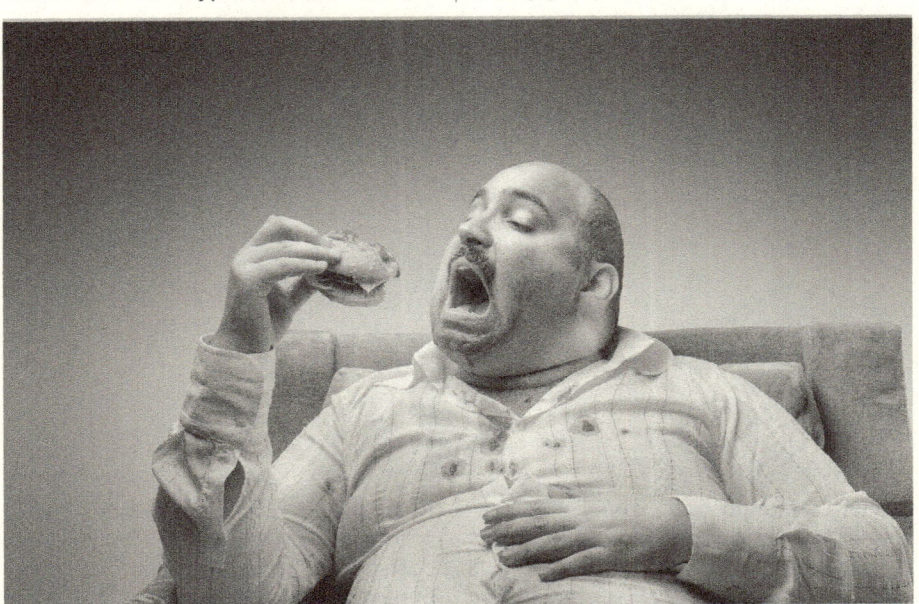

Regress When Required

Regression at appropriate times is an important part of progression, though this might sound counterintuitive. Regression means returning to a former or less developed state (for example, going back to a lower kettlebell weight, doing fewer reps, performing an easier exercise, etc.) Appropriate times for regression are when you're near fatigue, injured, not getting it, or need to perfect certain aspects of an exercise. For example, if you've progressed to snatching but after a few days find that you're having issues, you might want to regress back to swings. If you're having issues with your swing, you might need to regress back to the bodyweight hip hinge, and so on.

Regression is when you set your ego aside and think about your health in order to remain injury-free. When you're WODing, where the prescribed weight is

24kg, and you're going up against Tina and Mike who have been training for years, and swing those 24kg kettlebells like they're nothing, don't worry about how you look compared to them. Regress during the workout if you need to, and grab a lower weight. Tell the trainer you need to do fewer reps, or whatever you have to do to remain injury-free while still completing a successful workout.

What is Shoulder Packing?

If you completely relax your shoulders and have someone else move your upper arm around in any direction he/she pleases, it would move quite freely in and out of its socket. The goal is to prevent any instability in that area during weightlifting, so you want to provide stability by "packing" the shoulders. Not only does shoulder packing prevent injury, it also allows you to get stronger and lift more weight by providing a stable base to press or pull from.

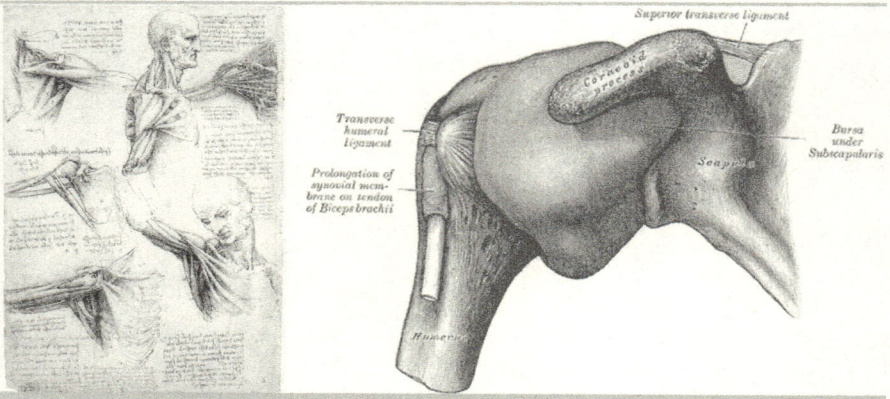

Here's how to do it: You pack your shoulders by pushing your chest out slightly, pulling your lats down, slightly squeezing the shoulder blades together while pulling the shoulder blades down and creating a firm chest. The desired position to achieve is the shoulders pressed down and away from the ears.

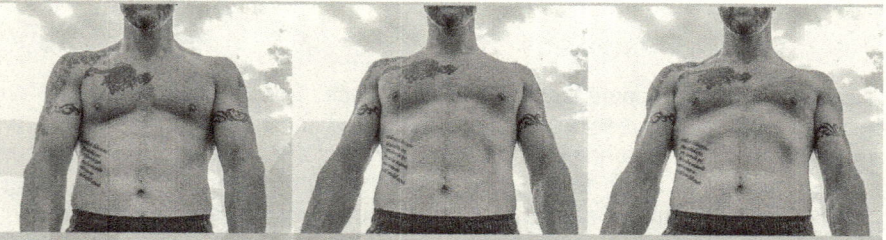

Normal. Back. Down.

You don't kick a soccer ball with a loose/relaxed knee or hip joint, do you?

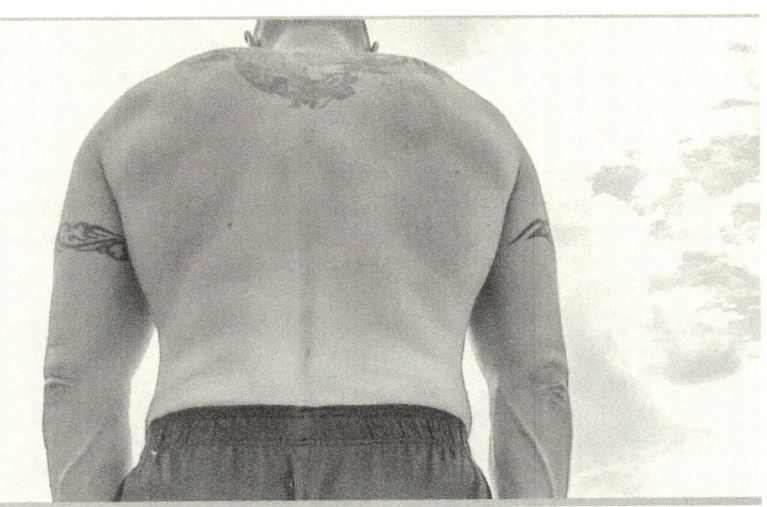

Normal.

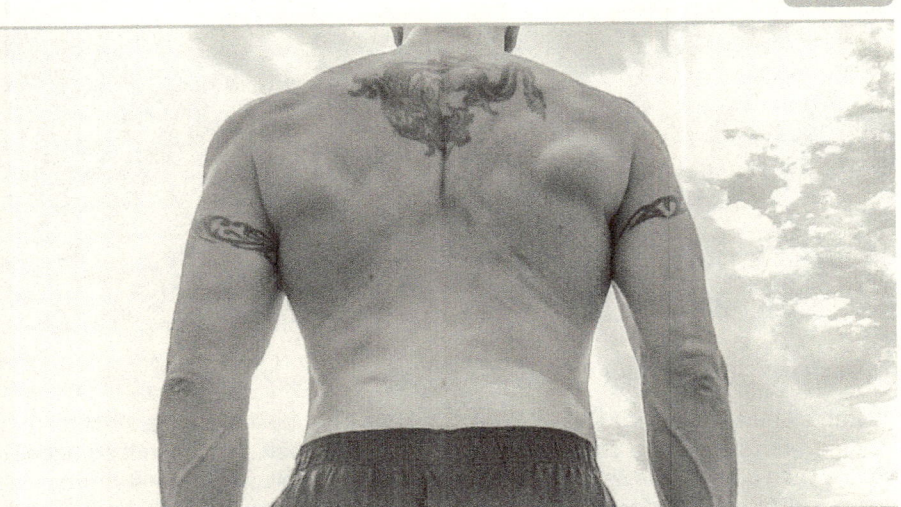

Back and down.

ARE KETTLEBELLS SAFE?

YES, KETTLEBELLS ARE EXTREMELY SAFE
within the proper context.

"Anyone who starts kettlebell training needs to follow the kettlebell journey step by step; they need to go through the rites of passage; there are no shortcuts."

Taco Fleur

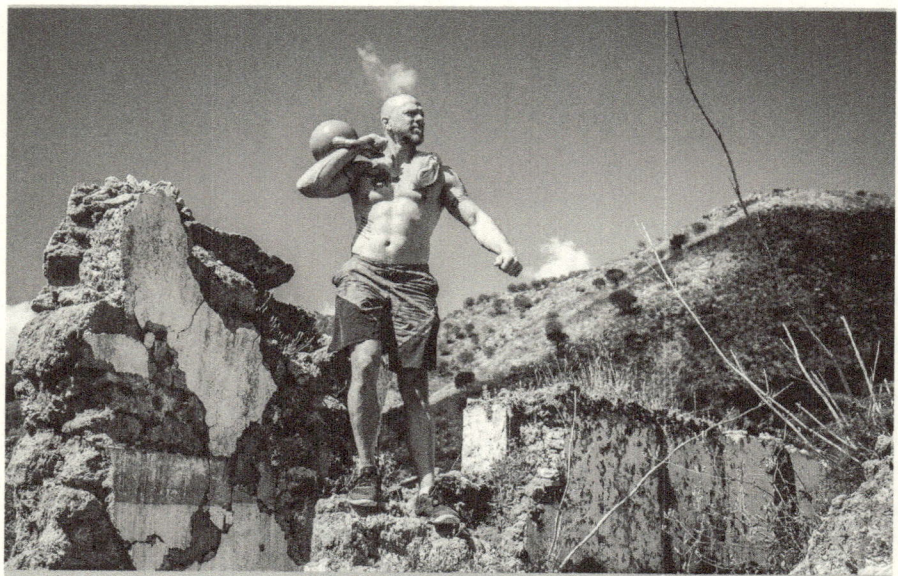

AVOID GETTING HURT

Grab a kettlebell in your first week of training and start doing snatches like you've seen other, more seasoned kettlebell enthusiasts perform with ease, and you're playing with fire. There is no doubt you're going to get hurt. The same applies to any other discipline; grab a barbell in your first week of training and start snatching it like you're in the CrossFit Games, you're going to get hurt!

This fact doesn't change whether using a dumbbell, TRX, sandbag, fitball, or anything else; you need to respect the tool and treat it with care. You'll need to progress from step one, just like starting at Level 1 as Mario on the Nintendo - you don't just start on Level 32 and take on Tutankoopa, just like you don't take on the kettlebell snatch from day one.

PROGRESSION IS KEY

Progression is a journey of taking your kettlebell training step by step, a journey preferably done with a certified kettlebell trainer. Don't get dragged into the "this style is better" trap – learn them all. You will usually start with the conventional double-arm swing, progress to single-arm swing, cleans, presses, Turkish get-ups, and snatches. There is a great deal more to learn in between, but that pace depends on your time, coach, and goals.

The way a coach furthers you all depends on your learning capabilities and goals. Some of these exercises might not mean anything to you yet; just know that the progression is from safely coming down, picking up the weight, lifting the weight, getting explosive with the weight, into more advanced exercises that build upon that basis.

Here is one way I might advance someone with online coaching from no experience to a professional kettlebell enthusiast, taking into consideration that the student has no injuries and is in good physical shape:

- Assessment
- Assisted single-arm clean
- Bodyweight squat
- Bodyweight hip hinge
- Kettlebell hang lift
- Kettlebell dead lift
- Dead clean
- Racking
- Conventional two-arm swing
- Two-arm clean
- Single-arm swing
- Single-arm swing clean
- Front squat
- Bent-over rows
- Strict press
- Push press
- Jerk
- Turkish get-up
- Snatch

An assessment will depend on the client's requirements and goals. If they're generic, the assessment will be standard and test everything: cardio, flexibility, strength, muscle endurance, and so on.

I cover the assisted single-arm clean very early, as I like my students to get familiar with the corkscrew motion and learning proper weight distribution of the kettlebell to avoid pressure on the forearm, which, if not dealt with early on, hinders progression at the stage of racking, cleaning, and pressing.

After those fundamental exercises, I would consider adding another arsenal of kettlebell exercises, grinding, rotational, explosive, etc.

PROGRESSION FOR BEGINNERS

Another great progression that I use for most beginners is as follows:

- Bodyweight hip hinge
- Kettlebell deadlift hip hinge style
- Assisted clean (Video youtube.com/watch?v=BniipxsR-BI)
- Racking
- Hang clean
- Dead clean (Video youtube.com/watch?v=vDk9buzo6BY)
- Double-arm swing (AKA Russian swing)
- Single arm swing (Video youtu.be/VCEWRgyHvHU)
- Alternating swing
- Swing clean
- Press (Video 50+ presses youtube.com/watch?v=svZhi3GHzKY)
- Rows (Video youtube.com/watch?v=WpK-4gjaKoI)
- High pull
- Snatch (Video youtube.com/watch?v=21cGGTGIUts)
- Overhead reverse lunge (Video youtube.com/watch?v=y6A8IKVEONQ)
- Windmill (Anyhow windmill video youtube.com/watch?v=P7JpZwMk8jo)
- Turkish get-up (Video youtube.com/watch?v=AYcKnpEusiw)

Many hundreds of kettlebell exercises to follow after this. Note that the progression is not always the same; it depends on the clients' goals, duration of training, and learning curve. Make sure you follow our Facebook group to stay up to date when we publish our new book, All Kettlebell Exercises, containing all the kettlebell exercises you can imagine.

FACEBOOK.COM/CAVEMANTRAINING

ARE KETTLEBELLS BAD FOR YOUR SHOULDERS?

If you start doing weird things that you should not be doing, or your body is just not ready for this type of exercise, kettlebells can be bad for your shoulders like any other body part; however, used appropriately they're amazing for shaping your shoulders, creating a better range of motion, and making shoulders stronger and more resilient to injury.

ARE KETTLEBELLS BAD FOR YOUR BACK?

That's like asking "are bicep curls bad for your biceps?". Kettlebells are the perfect tool to help eradicate chronic back pain, but again, only when done right. The people that ask these questions either have participated in a kettlebell class with a cowboy trainer or might have heard grumbles from a friend who just started swinging around after watching a Jillian Michaels version of the swing on YouTube and began to complain about their back.

If I said I had never seen anyone get injured during kettlebell training, that would be a lie. I have not, however, seen serious injury from a kettlebell when used correctly. I have seen people out for a week, because they did not listen to the suggested weight; they did not listen when the coach said to take a step back, regress and learn the hip hinge first. What I do know is that I've seen far fewer injuries in kettlebell training than any other form of training. I believe this is largely due to the unilateral qualities of the kettlebell, which leads me to my favourite saying:

> *"Press a 40kg barbell and your dominant side will usually press more, but press two twenties, and you're pressing two twenties!"*
> **Taco Fleur**

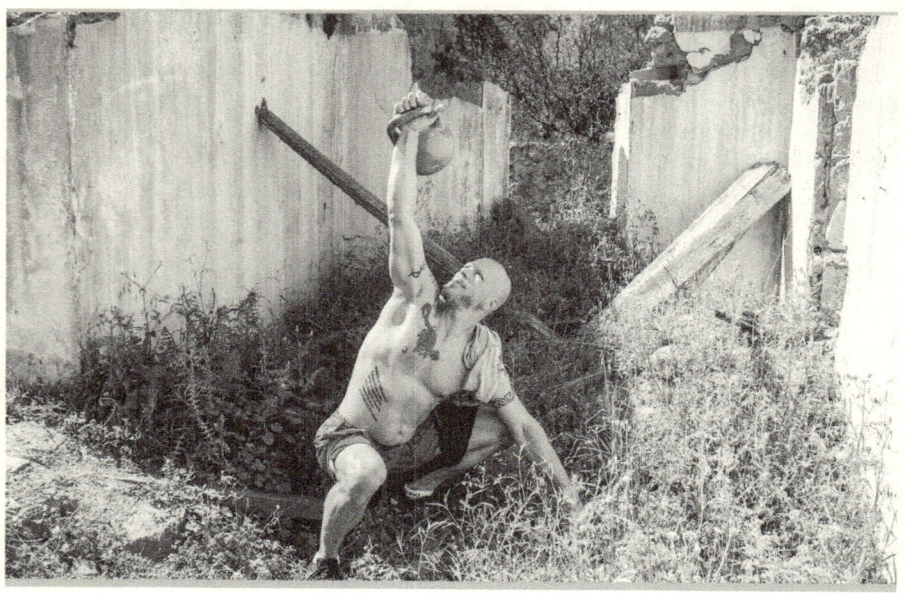

Respect the tools, follow the progression, and use common sense. Learn everything you can, but keep only what works for you. Kettlebells are as safe to use as YOU make them. Learn the basics, learn good form, and advance slowly.

WARMING UP FOR KETTLEBELL TRAINING

Kettlebell training is a type of training that always adds resistance to the workout; a kettlebell workout is never done with bodyweight alone; therefore a proper warm-up is always required.

There is no "one size fits all" warm-up that can be used for all kettlebell workouts; however, some aspects remain the same across all warm-ups:

- Preferably utilize bodyweight for the warm-up
- Warm-up and prepare the whole body for exercise
- Focus more on the areas of the body that will be utilized during the workout
- Mimic exercises with bodyweight that will be performed in the workout
- Include dynamic but not static stretching
- Slowly and gradually increase the intensity of a warm-up
- Slowly and gradually increase complexity

Although a good warm-up is important for everyone, it's even more important for unconditioned people, as it helps avoid a rapid increase in blood pressure.

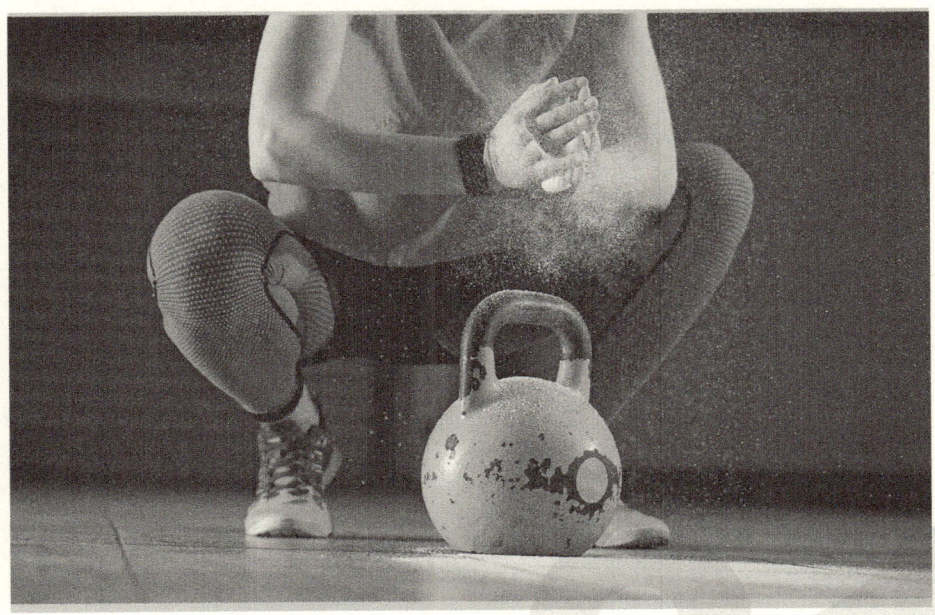

WHY WARM-UP?

- ✓ Injury prevention
- ✓ Mental preparation for the workout
- ✓ Increase the heart-rate to increase oxygen-rich blood flow to working muscles
- ✓ To gently stretch the muscles before working out
- ✓ Release synovial fluid to loosen the joints and reduce friction during movement
- ✓ Prompt hormonal changes in the body responsible for regulating energy production
- ✓ Reduce potential aches and pains
- ✓ Muscles that are not properly warmed up do not absorb shock or impact as well

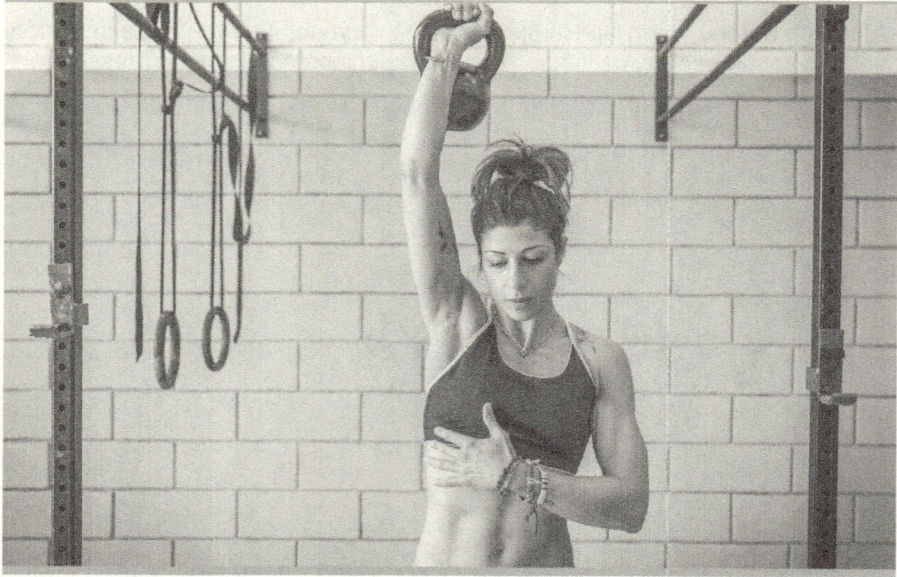

FOCUS

Although you should always prepare the whole body for exercise, there are times when workouts are more upper-body or lower-body concentrated, and in that case the warm-up should focus more on that area, while not neglecting other areas.

MIMIC THE WORKOUT

It's always a good idea to mimic the exercises that will be performed in the workout. For example, if you're doing a kettlebell windmill in your workout, then you want to include the bodyweight windmill in your warm-up, and perform more rotational bodyweight exercises; if you're doing a Turkish get-up in your workout then you want to include the bodyweight TGU and lunges; if you're doing front squats, include the bodyweight squat. All of these examples mirror or target the exercises included in the workout.

Good mornings and bodyweight hip hinges are great for when the workout includes kettlebell swings, as they either work the same muscle groups or mimic the same movement, but without resistance.

WHY INCREASE THE TEMPERATURE?

Increasing the temperature of the muscles is good, because your muscles need oxygen to function. At a higher temperature, the haemoglobin in your blood releases oxygen more readily, and your muscles are also able to contract and relax at a faster pace, which all attributes to a better and enhanced performance.

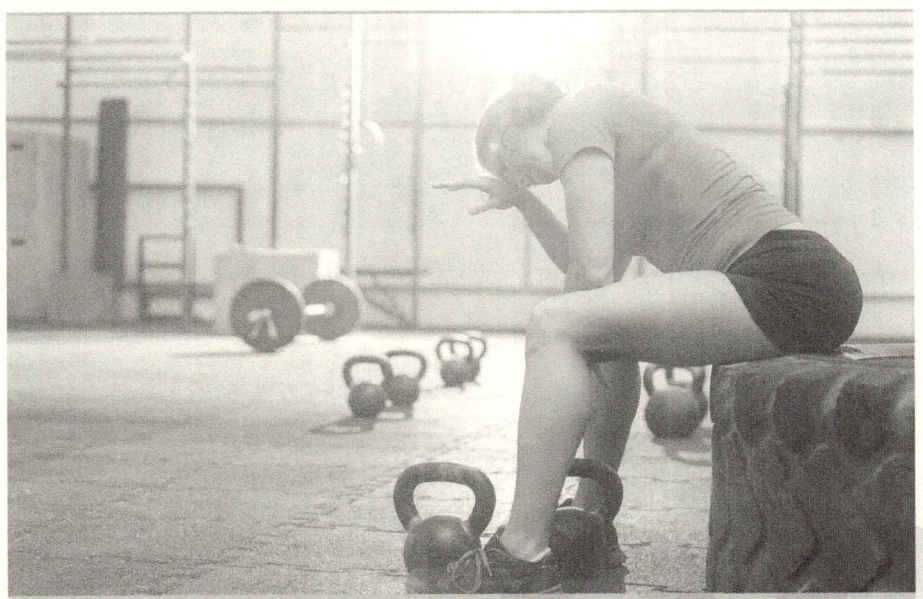

WHY INCREASE THE BLOOD FLOW?

After 10 to 12 minutes of total body exercise, blood flow to the skeletal muscles increases to some 70 to 75 percent, and the capillaries open, enabling more blood, and hence oxygen to be available to working muscles.

DURATION

Although there is no magic number which works for each and every workout, a good duration is anywhere between 5 to 10 minutes or longer for unconditioned people. The more resistance is added to the workout, the longer the warm-up should be; for a full bodyweight work-out one could drastically reduce the duration of the warm-up.

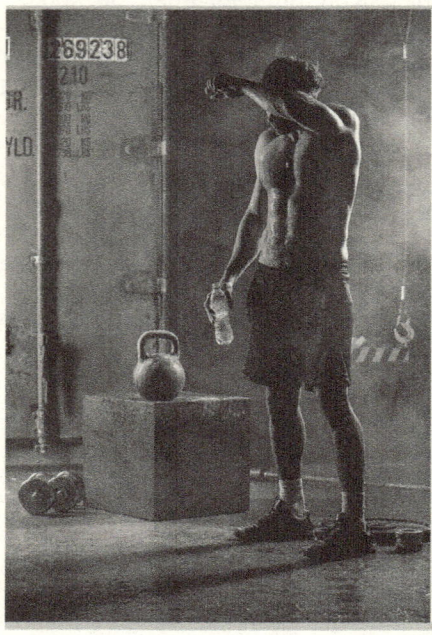
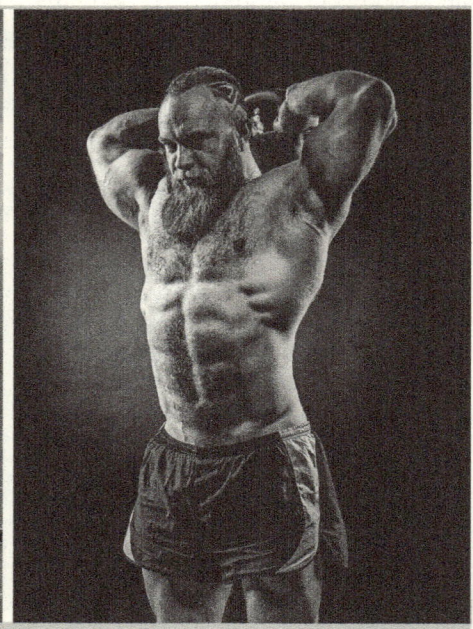

INCREASE OF INTENSITY AND COMPLEXITY

The following is an example of a lower-body warm-up that gradually increases intensity and complexity. Due to the hip hinge and good mornings, this would be a good candidate as a warm-up for kettlebell swings:

- 30s slow paced high knees
- 30s half hip hinge
- 30s slow paced half squat
- 30s good morning
- 10s quick feet

- 30s hip hinge
- 30s deep squat
- 10s quick feet
- 20s squat jumps
- 10s quick feet

Following is an example of an upper-body warm-up that gradually increases intensity and complexity. Due to the push-ups, this would be a good candidate as a warm-up for the kettlebell chest press:

- 15s shoulder rolls forwards
- 15s shoulder rolls backwards youtube.com/watch?v=-g91PZvVad0
- 20s one arm up, one arm down and alternate youtube.com/watch?v=g7-jSx-74Ilo
- 30s jumping jacks youtu.be/xE6SZP9kkmc?t=15s
- 15s chest push-ups
- 15s tricep push-ups
- 20s arms in and out (hug yourself, open up the chest, and pull the shoulder blades together) youtube.com/watch?v=gUyRAtuG_Kc
- 30s jumping jacks
- 30s chest push-ups
- 30s tricep push-ups

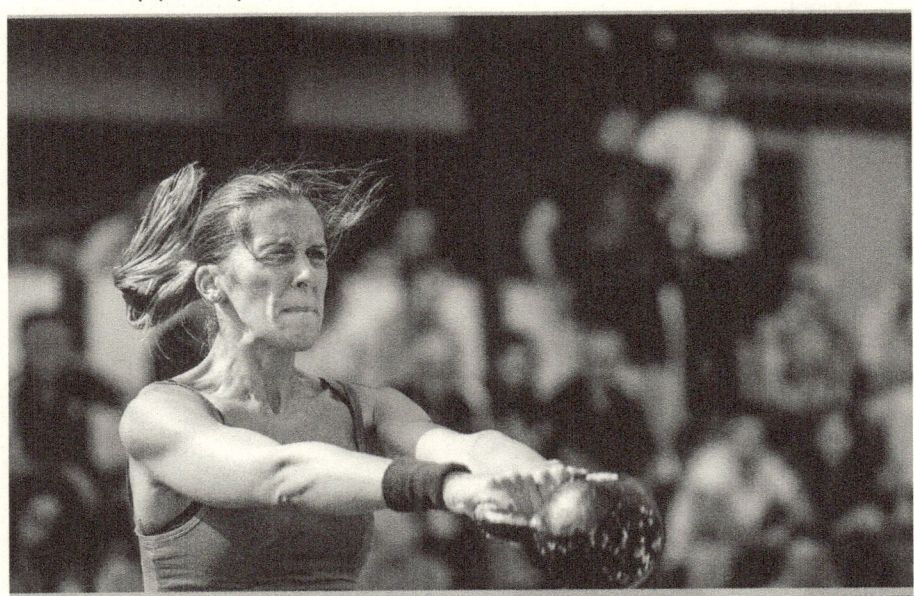

WHICH KETTLEBELL TO CHOOSE AND WHY?

I'm a great advocate for competition kettlebells, even when not used for Kettlebell Sport. That said, I'll provide as much information about the different kettlebells available, so you can make your own decision.

If you're just starting out with kettlebell training, you'll want to start with something light, so that you can focus on form and technique. Starting out with a weight that is too heavy will compromise your form and technique, and potentially cause injury.

Differences:

- ✔ Handle diameter
- ✔ Handle shape
- ✔ Window diameter
- ✔ Base diameter
- ✔ Bell dimension
- ✔ Weight
- ✔ Colour
    - Coat
    - Neoprene
    - Rubber
    - Vinyl
    - Powder
- ✔ Material
    - Steel
    - Iron
- ✔ Filling
    - Sand
    - Water
    - Hollow

Competition Kettlebells AKA Pro Grade Kettlebells, Sport Kettlebells, Girya Sport Kettlebell

Classic Kettlebells AKA Iron-cast Kettlebells

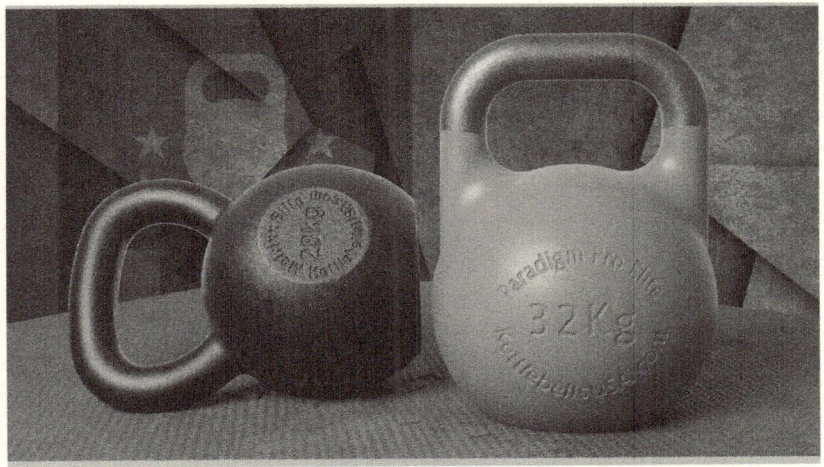

Cast-iron versus Steel Competition Kettlebell

Classic Kettlebells are less expensive than the Competition Kettlebells.

As mentioned earlier, my preference is the Competition Kettlebell and the reason for that is the competition kettlebell remains the same size, no matter what weight you work with; whether it's an 8kg or 24kg, the size of the kettlebell remains the same. This is a great feature, because there is no need to get used to different shapes and sizes when you go up in weight. Furthermore, the base of the comp kettlebell is a lot wider, allowing you to do things like burpee deadlifts, renegade rows, and other exercises where you need to place your weight on the kettlebell - a narrow base has the potential for the bell to topple over and cause wrist injury. I personally find it difficult to find comfortable positions with the classic kettlebells, especially the lighter weight.

Rubber, neoprene, and vinyl coated kettlebells are more suitable for surfaces that scratch or chip easy. Vinyl is harder and more resistant to damage than rubber. Neoprene is softer than both rubber and vinyl, which increases comfort. All that said, I've not had good experience with these type of coated kettlebells myself.

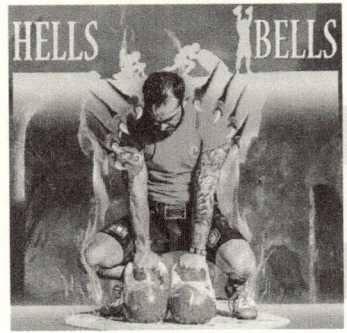

David Keohan

International Kettlebell Colour Standard for Competition Kettlebells:

Weight in Kilos	Weight in Pounds	Colour
8	17.6	Pink
12	26.4	Blue
16	35.2	Yellow
20	44.0	Purple
24	52.8	Green
28	61.6	Orange
32	70.4	Red
36	79.2	Grey
40	88.0	White
44	96.8	Silver
48	105.6	Gold

There are also weights in between (for example, 10 kg, 14 kg, and so on), and these are usually coloured with a different shade of the neighbouring weight, or defined by a black band on the handle.

WHAT WEIGHT TO CHOOSE?

The weight you choose for training depends on your goals and what exercises you will primarily be doing with it, in addition to your current strength. If we're talking primarily about double-arm swings done by absolute beginners, I'd suggest 8kg or less for children, 10kg to 12kg for adolescents, 12kg for women, and 14 to 16kg for men.

For overhead pressing, I suggest at least 4 to 6kg less than mentioned for the swings above. For chest pressing, 2 to 4kg less, as most people are stronger with chest presses compared to overhead presses.

For rowing with the focus being on the rear deltoids, I suggest the same weight as for swings or even slightly more weight. For rows that focus more on the middle of the back, I suggest the same weight as for overhead presses.

For deadlifts, squat style, I suggest the same as swings or more, and possibly even double kettlebells. For deadlifts hip hinge, I recommend the same as swings or slightly less.

That covers the basic exercises. If you're talking about any other exercise, you've already progressed and are more than likely able to make an informed decision on what weight to use.

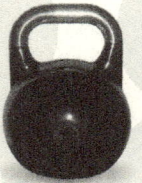 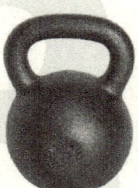 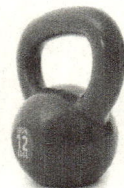 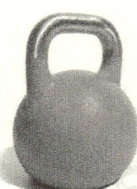

Where to Buy Kettlebells Online

Out of the many places to buy kettlebells online, you'll see the following names and brands pop up the most: Amazon, Onnit, Agatsu, Ader, Kettlebells USA, Kettlebell Kings, Dragon-Door Kettlebells.

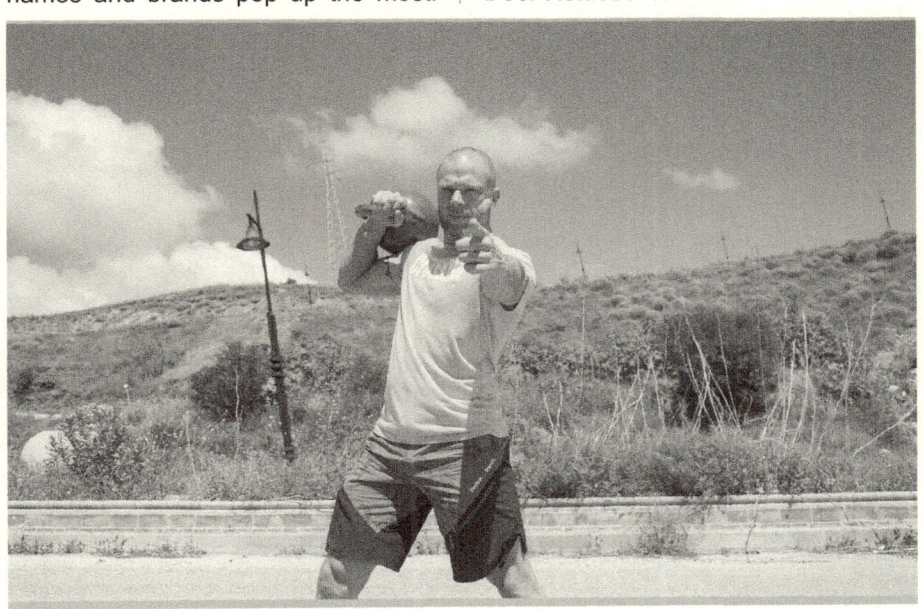

KETTLEBELL GRIPS

Details on kettlebell grips are often neglected in courses and books; however, grips are fundamental, and can make a world of difference between comfort, efficiency, and injury. Definitions of grip:

Grip /grip/: verb

1. Take and keep a firm hold of; grasp tightly
2. A firm hold; a tight grasp or clasp
3. A part or attachment by which something is held in the hand

There are many different types of kettlebell grips you will need to employ during kettlebell training; following are illustrations and basic explanations of what each different grip is used for. If you enrolled in one of our free or paid online kettlebell courses, you will see references to these different grips.

Important: With each grip there are only one or two exercises listed to get the general idea across, but in most cases there are many more than those listed. Grips might differ slightly across kettlebells as the width of the handle increases with some of the classic kettlebells when the weight goes up.

Along your kettlebell journey, you will find that different associations or organizations will use different grips for different exercises, and as long as it works and is safe, there is nothing wrong with that.

For illustration purposes, a competition kettlebell is used, which changes in weight but not in size.

Note that these are **not** barbell grips; the names might be the same, but the technique is not.

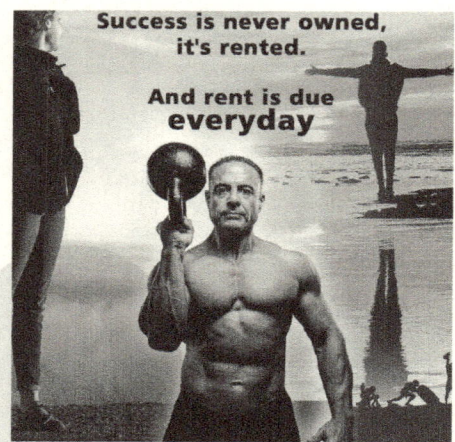

Shawn Powers

GENERAL GRIP INFORMATION

The following few basic rules and tips apply to most kettlebell grips.

A grip on the kettlebell handle or horns should almost never be tight; it should always be as loose as possible without losing grip on the kettlebell and conserving as much grip strength without burning out the muscles.

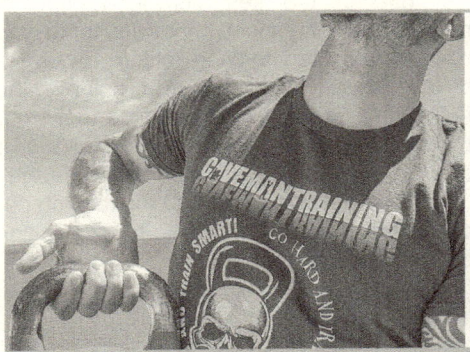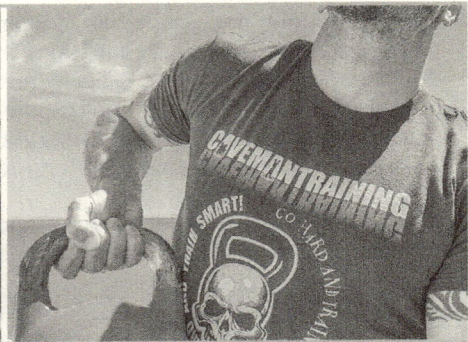

Loose versus tight grip

Blisters usually occur when the skin is folded within the grip, especially when using heavy weights or doing high-volume reps. Try to slide your fingers around the handle or horns while avoiding skin folds from occurring, and then close the grip. Another cause for blisters is friction; avoid friction by proper kettlebell guidance.

Ripped calluses occur when there is friction within the palms, and the biggest culprit is kettlebell bobbing. To prevent the kettlebell from bobbing at the end of the down phase, you want to be inserting the kettlebell between the legs rather completing a full pendulum.

The most common grip and transition is from hook grip to loose grip, which occurs during the clean and rack. The hook grip is also used for single arm swings and snatches; the second most common grip is the double hand grip, which is used for double arm swings.

These are just a few tips and fundamentals to get you going with an effective grip on the kettlebell.

WHY SHOULD YOU LEARN ABOUT GRIPS?

It is important to know and understand kettlebell grips for efficiency and being able to work the muscles intended for the exercise in question. Employing an incorrect grip can cause pain, discomfort, inefficiency, injury, and exhaustion of grip, forearm, biceps, or shoulder muscles, as well as losing focus on the muscles targeted within a specific exercise.

WHY USE DIFFERENT GRIPS?

If you're asking this question, then you're on the right track. Knowing a lot of grips is cool, but knowing why you would change grip or use one over the other is even cooler, and the part you should really understand.

During kettlebell training, you employ different grips to make certain exercises more efficient, but you also change grips to increase difficulty and challenge other muscle groups. Sometimes when your training gets stale you might even employ a different grip to entertain the mind.

While knowing kettlebell grips and when to employ them is important and one of the kettlebell fundamentals, the second most important thing you should start looking into is racking a kettlebell. It might seem insignificant, but a lot hinges on how you rack your kettlebell; in fact, some people give up on kettlebell training, because they can't get comfortable in the racking position, or can't find the proper position for the bell to rest.

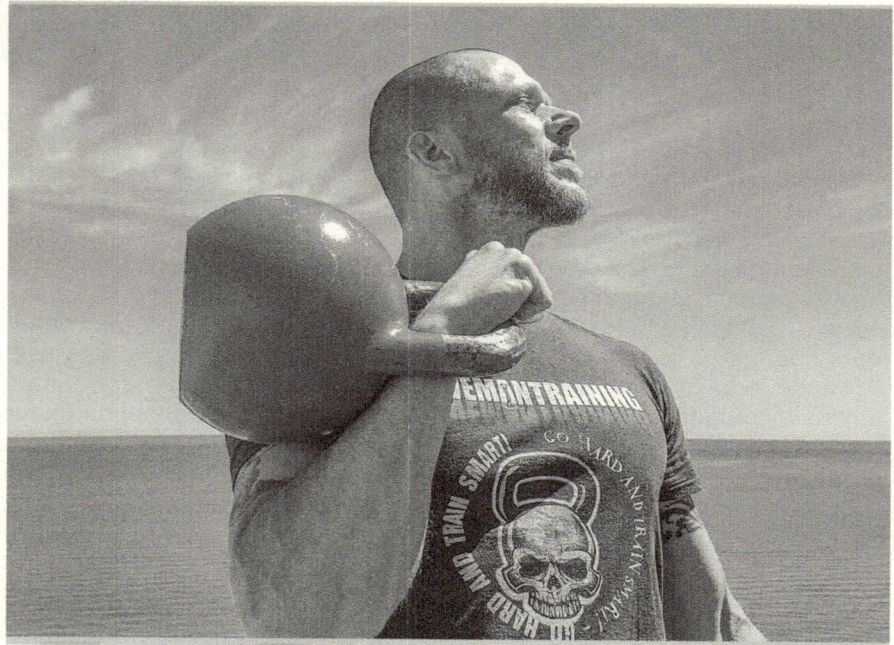

ANATOMY OF THE KETTLEBELL

The following illustration breaks down the anatomy of the kettlebell. Knowing the exact names for parts of the kettlebell will help you understand given instructions better and increase clarity when teaching kettlebell training.

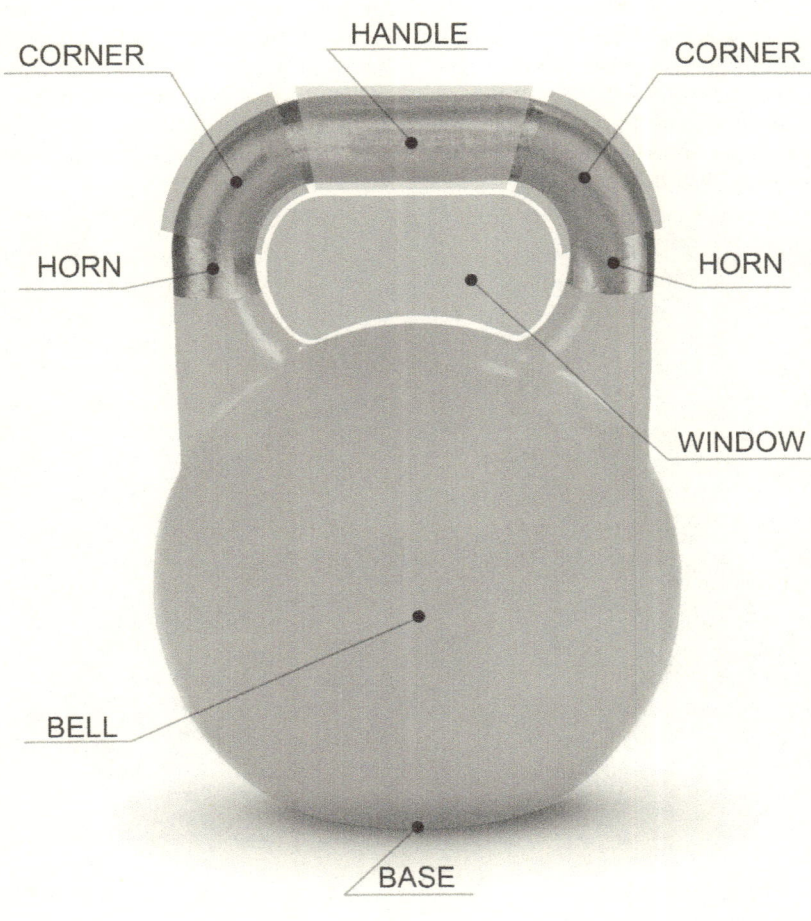

- Handle
- Horn(s)
- Corner(s)
- Window
- Bell
- Base

HAND POSITION ON THE HANDLE

Your hand position changes depending on what exercise you're going to do (i.e., your hand position on the handle will be different if you're doing single arm swings as opposed to swings mixed with cleans). Your hand position will be different if you're doing sport style snatches or hard style. If you're doing single arm swings, you may want to hold the handle in the middle for even weight distribution.

At times, the hand position is dictated by preference. Some might have perfected sliding from the middle to the corner and have a personal reason for doing so. What you need to know is that there is a reason to place your hand correctly on the handle; be aware of what positions are available, and learn the most common techniques first, then adjust to your own style as you progress.

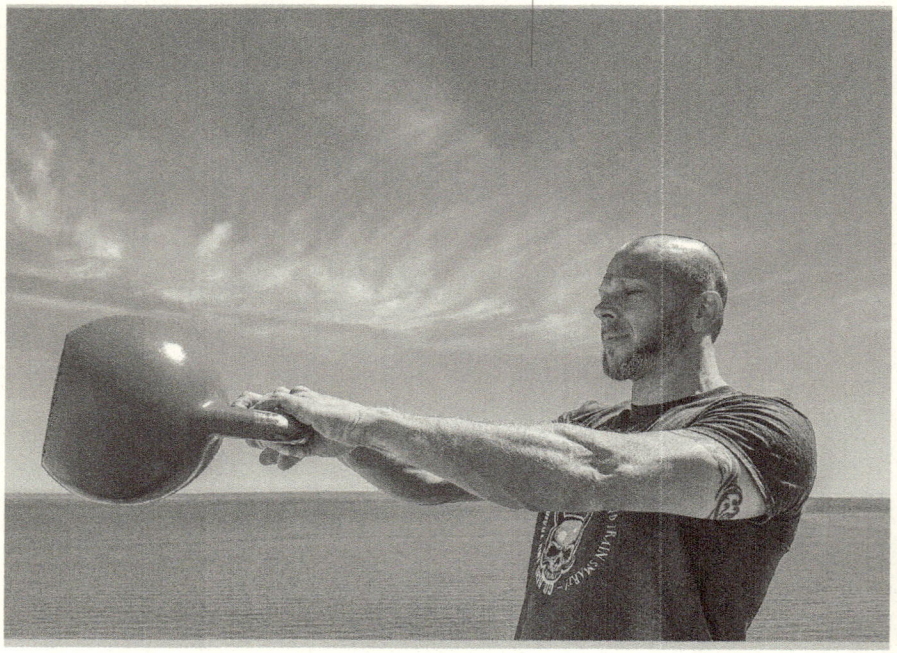

Most common grip, double hand grip for the conventional kettlebell swing

45 DEGREE ANGLE

In grips employed for racking or pressing, the handle should be positioned at a 45 degree angle within the palm, one corner positioned on the webbing between the thumb and index finger, and the other corner being past the heel of the palm. The reason for this position is to keep the wrist straight and hand in line with the forearm, thus avoiding pressure on the wrist. A bent wrist means there is a kink in the line through which power will be lost during pressing and could cause injury.

When working with a light kettlebell, this might not be as noticeable, but when working with heavier kettlebells the pressure can be enormous, causing damage to the wrist and/or preventing you from being able to press the kettlebell up.

When people first start training with a kettlebell, you'll find that they employ the 'broken wrist grip' to relieve the pressure that the bell puts on the forearm; this is especially true for new people who are not used to this pressure. Trainers should take the person aside and have him/her play with the grip, handle position, and bell positioning till they feel comfortable with the pressure of the kettlebell being in the correct position. It's also helpful to explain that it's quite normal to experience some mild discomfort until the area is more conditioned.

See photos below for correct 45 degree handle angle in the palm.

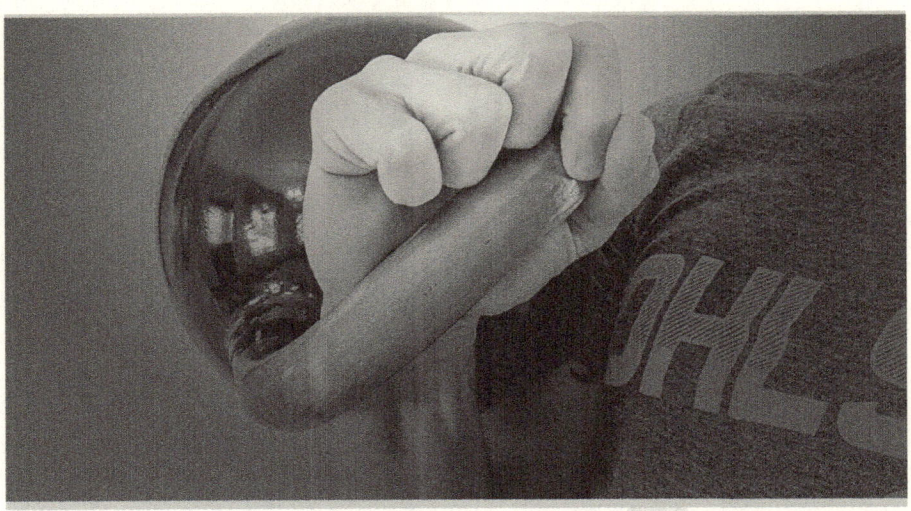

Correct 45° angle of the handle within the palm

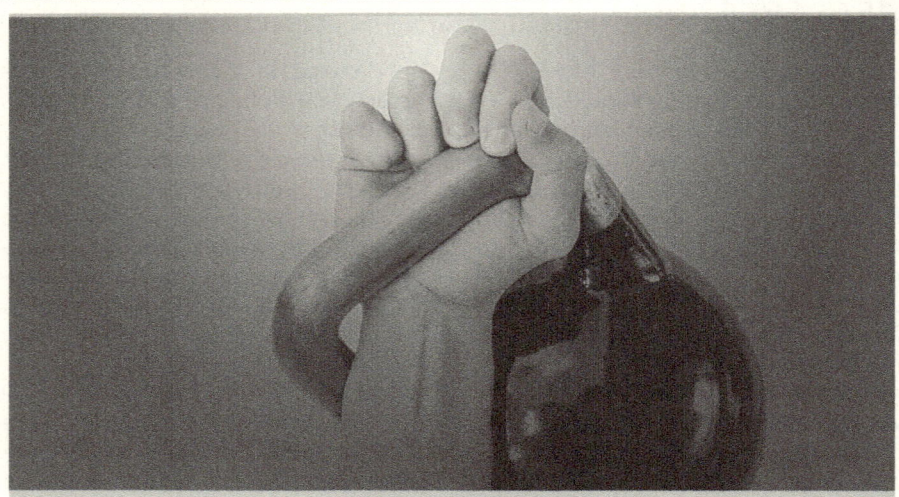

Correct 45° angle of the handle within the palm

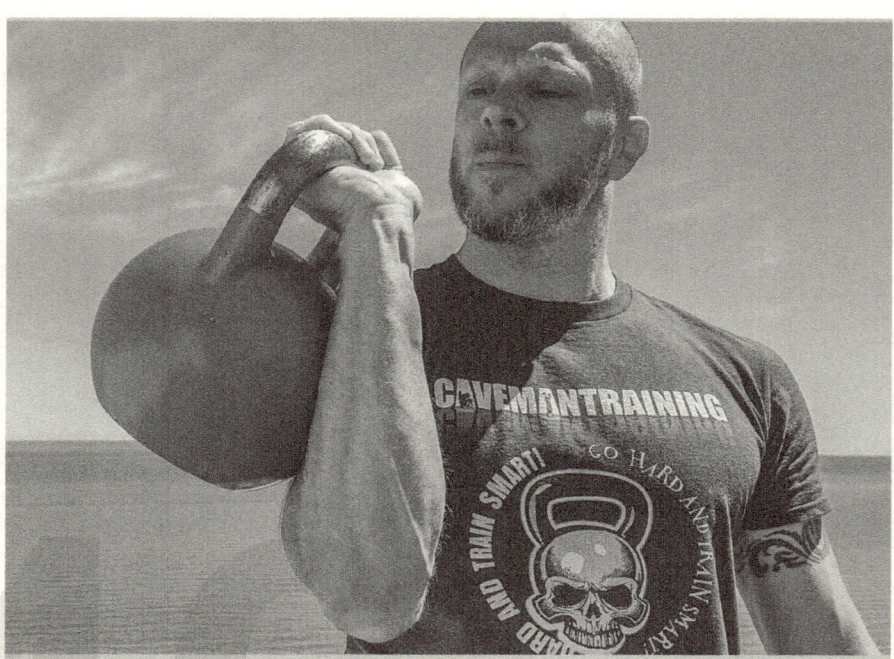

Handle incorrectly positioned within the palm, AKA "broken wrist" - note that the visible corner is not over the heel of the palm

GRIP CATEGORIES

Grips can be categorized as follows:
- Pressing grips
- Racking grips
- Lifting grips
- Ballistic grips
- Juggling grips

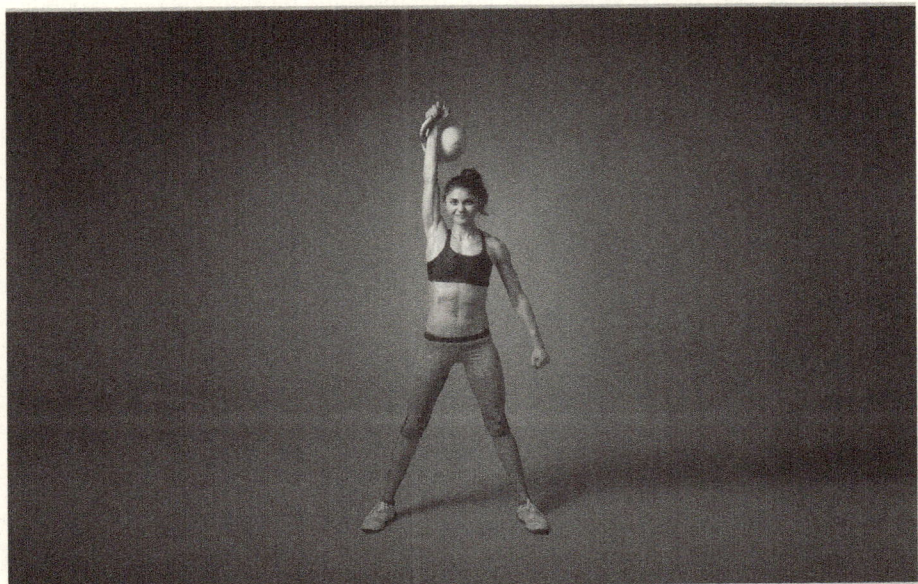

DOUBLE HAND GRIP

Grip: two hands, four fingers closed around the handle placed on the corners or horns depending on hand size and thumbs loose.

Ideal for: double-arm swings and deadlifts

This grip is mostly used for doing double arm swings and deadlifts. Like with most grips, do not turn this into a tight grip; keep some space for the handle to move freely without causing friction. This grip should loosen up at the top part of the swing to stop the grip from burning out. You will have eight fingers around the handle. Those with big fingers might feel squashed when doing high volume reps, so pay particular attention to the ring fingers at high volume reps, as they are prone to blisters.

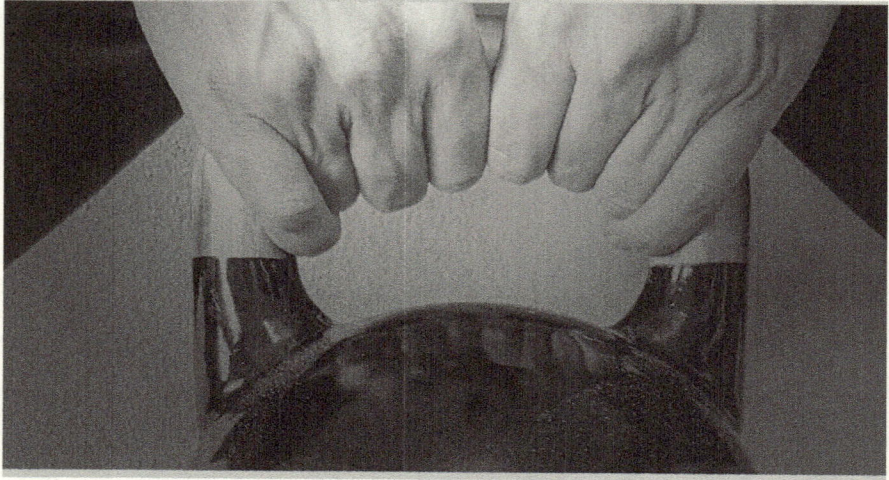

The grip can be employed with both of the pinkies positioned within the horns (pictured above) or over the horns (pictured further below under the Closed Double Hand Grip).

Following two grips are provided **by Valerie Pawlowski** *World Champion Kettlebe*

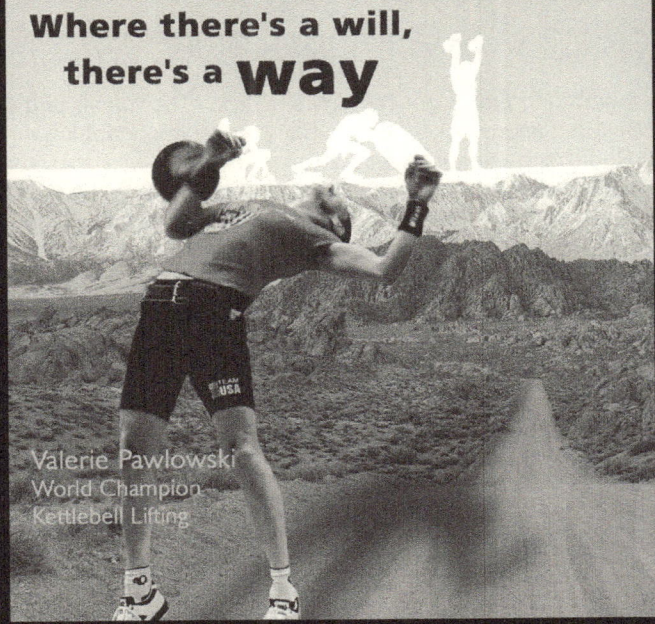

SWAN GRIP

This grip is used primarily in rowing drills and pulling or front-holding movements.

Grasping with fingers mostly straight in a beak-like hold over top of kettlebell, with arm bent at wrist and elbow in "S-like" position like that of a swan neck, with emphasis on squeeze of fingers and strong forearm engagement; this grip gives tremendous grip strength for massive finger and forearm recruitment.

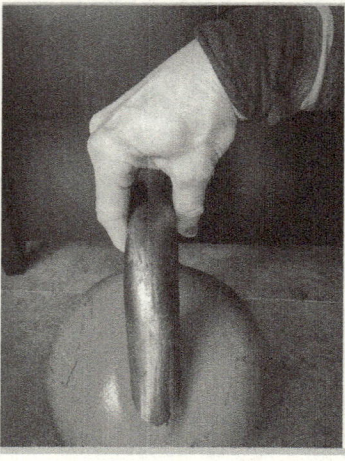
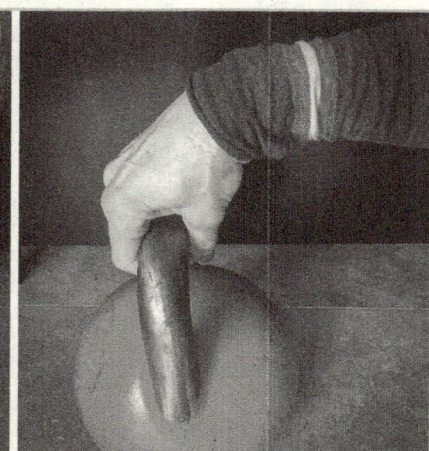

Swan grip

OK GRIP (AKA 2 OR 3 FINGER GRIP)

With thumb and first finger (and middle for 3) in a 2-finger lock wrap around handle. Remaining 3 fingers are off or relaxed (2 off on the ok 3 hold) away from handle.

Useful for carries, swings, clean, or row. The thumb and first finger are the most important to primary grip strength. Working with these variations puts attention on the longer lasting strength to hang on to the fullest extent, especially digging out on final snatches.

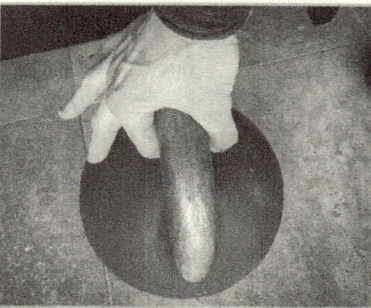
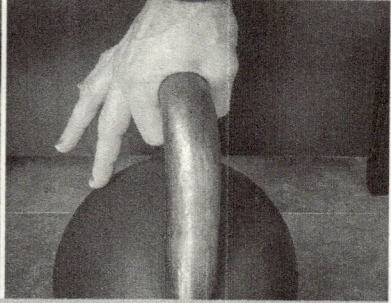

OK Grip - with thanks to Valerie Pawlowski for the photos and information.

CORKSCREW GRIP

Grip: Same as the double hand grip but with the horns between the pinkie and ring fingers.

Ideal for: double-arm swings and American swings

This is a grip I started using when doing heavy high-volume swings during the Cavemantraining 28-Day Kettlebell Swing Challenge, which I like to call the Double Hand Corkscrew Grip, because it's very similar to a grip on a corkscrew.

When holding a corkscrew, the screw itself will be positioned between the middle finger and ring finger, but with the kettlebell the horn will be positioned between the ring finger and pinkie. Everything from the Double Hand Grip transfers to this grip. I like to use this grip to switch it up, but also because I have big hands and usually need to put my pinkies over the handles with the Double Hand Grip.

With this grip, I feel that my fingers are less squashed. It is very important to wrap your pinkies around the horn to prevent them from getting caught in your clothes during the swing. This grip also provides more stability at the top of the American Swing and helps prevent skin tears on the outside of the pinkie.

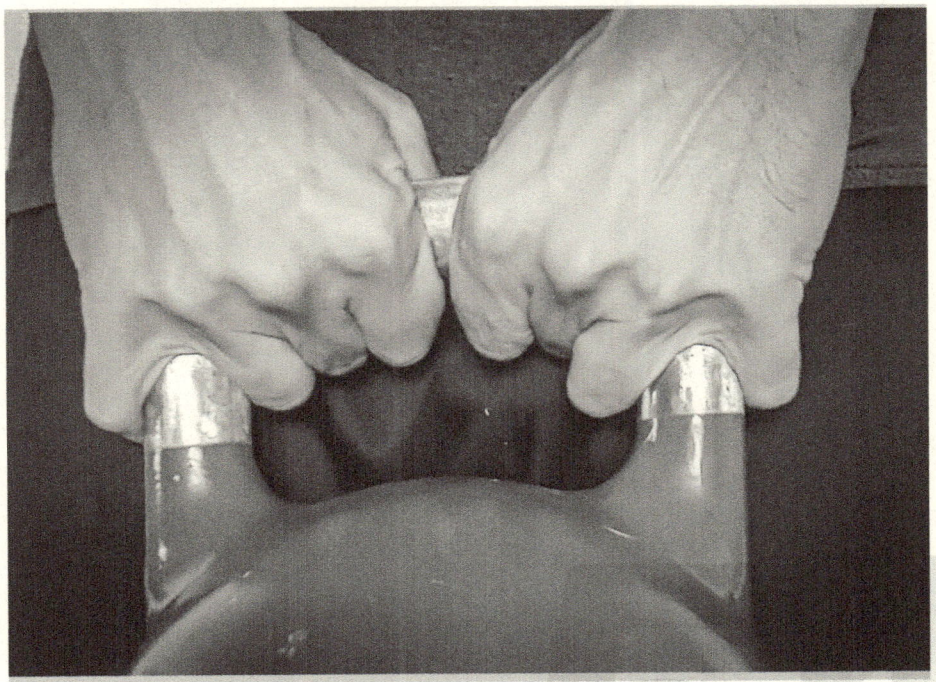

*Double hand **corkscrew** grip*

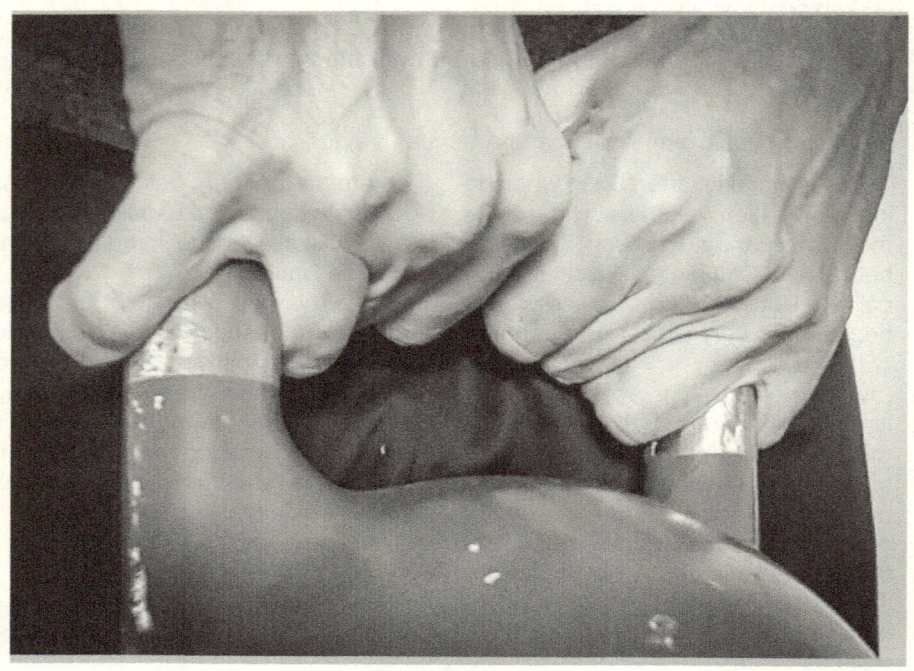

Double hand corkscrew grip

CLOSED DOUBLE HAND GRIP

Handle: two hands, four fingers and thumbs locking the index finger down, or locking both the index and middle finger down. Can also be with the pinkies over the horns as illustrated below, in which case it becomes three fingers plus lock.

Ideal for: double-arm swings, deadlifts

Everything from the Double Hand Grip transfers to this grip; the difference is that the thumbs are locking over the index fingers. This grip is for using extremely heavy weights, or high-volume swings when the grip is giving up. The lock is also employed to relieve some tension from the forearms. The lock might also be possible with one thumb two fingers. Note: This grip might not be possible with thicker handles.

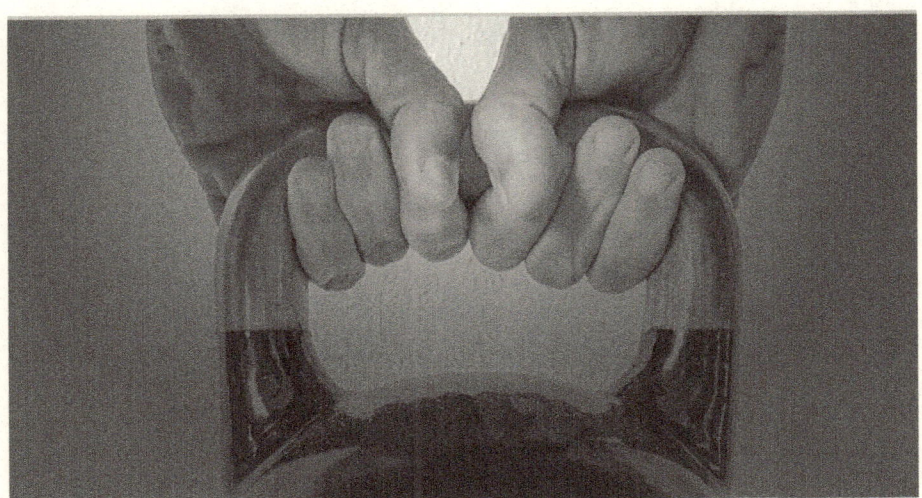

HOOK GRIP (AKA OVERHAND GRIP)

Handle: one hand, four fingers and thumb loose

Ideal for: down-phase of most ballistic movements, dead clean

With this grip, the handle is positioned within the fingers which are bent. It's used when the kettlebell travels downward for single arm swings and downward phase of snatches. Note that the thumb can move over to the other side of the handle (but not locking finger) and the hand is positioned closer to one side of the handle.

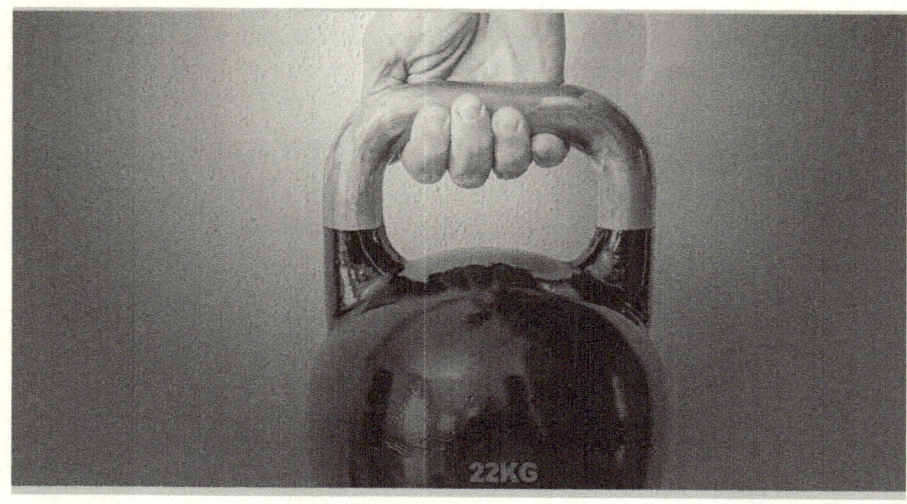

CLOSED HOOK GRIP (AKA C GRIP)

Handle: one hand, four fingers and thumb locking the index finger down, or both the index and middle finger

Ideal for: single-arm swings, snatch, dead clean

This grip is the same as the Hook Grip, apart from there being a finger lock with the thumb over forefinger. The lock provides a better grip but also serves to release tension on the forearms and fingers. If you experience finger cramps, forearm pain, or soreness, try switching to a closed hook grip. Issues arise primarily when just starting out with training or when doing high-volume reps without implementing a closed grip.

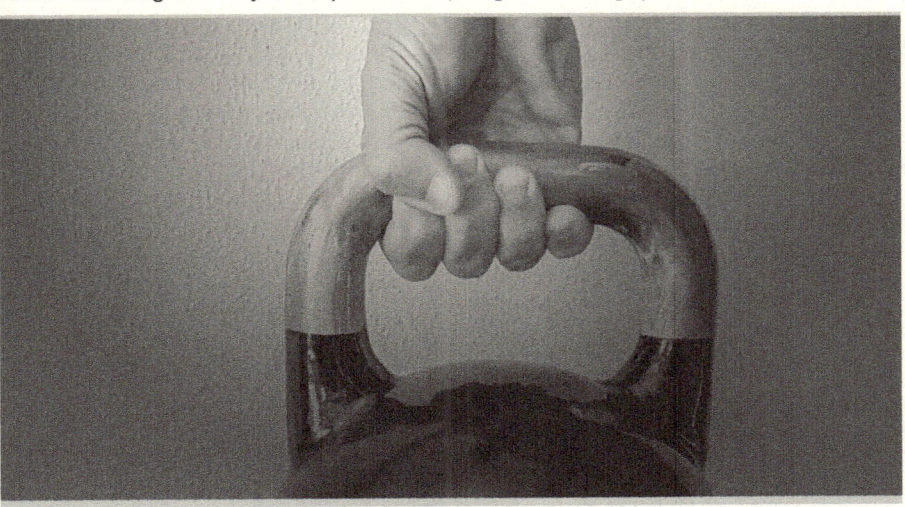

WHY USE HOOK GRIP?

If you're training with barbells, you're probably already familiar with the hook grip, but you should know that the hook grip is different in kettlebell training. I mention this because I've heard, "That's not a hook grip", pointed out to me plenty of times. In CrossFit, the hook grip is executed with the thumb over the bar and the fingers closing the grip over the thumb. In kettlebell training there is the Hook Grip and Closed Hook Grip (AKA C Grip) and the thumb is over the index finger or both the index and middle finger.

The hook grip is used to not only get a better, firmer grip on the bar or handle, but also to relieve some tension on your forearms. If you are experiencing finger cramps, tight forearms, muscle soreness, or other issues in your forearms, try switching to a hook grip. This is especially true when just starting training; your forearms and fingers still need to be conditioned.

Forearm flexors are located on the palm side of your forearm; you use these muscles when you curl, grip or hold things.

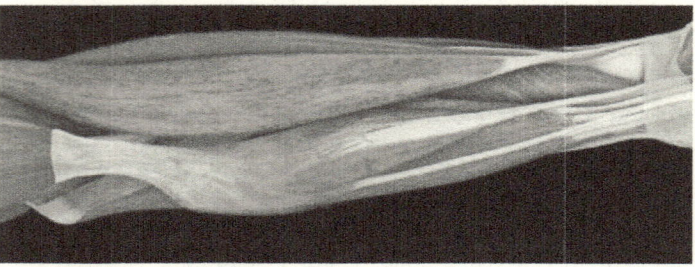

The function of the muscles in the forearms is to close the fingers into a fist or closed grip and keep them closed. While holding a weight, the barbell or kettlebell creates a constant tension on the muscles, and when not conditioned or doing high-volume reps this can turn into injury.

A closed hook grip or hook grip relieves some of the tension from the forearms, and furthermore, it involves the index finger more in the grip. Usually the index finger doesn't play a big role in the grip; you'll notice this when looking at the calluses on your palms.

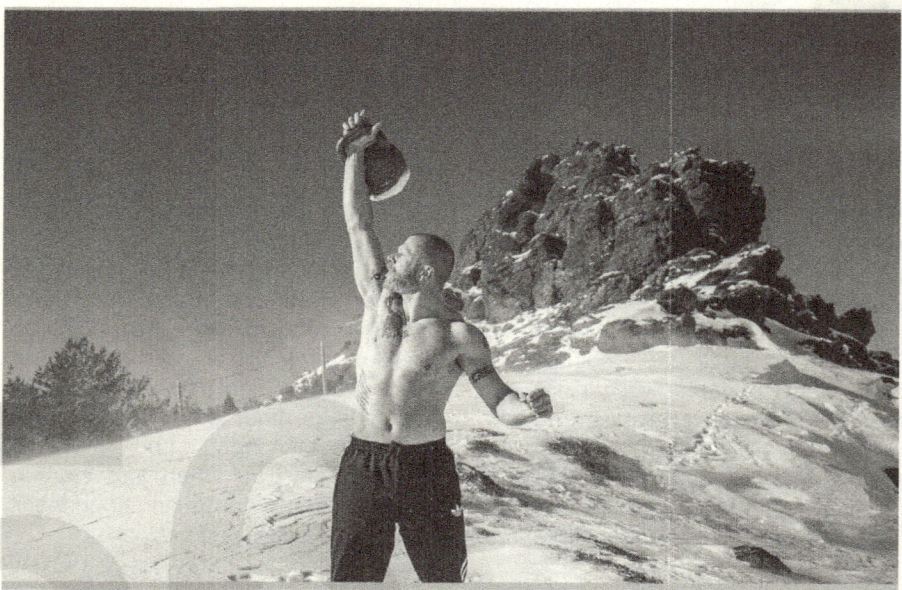

RACKING GRIP

This is the common grip employed in racking position with a closed but relaxed fist, fingers gently resting on the handle. If you work with two kettlebells, you should look at employing the Racking Safety Grip.

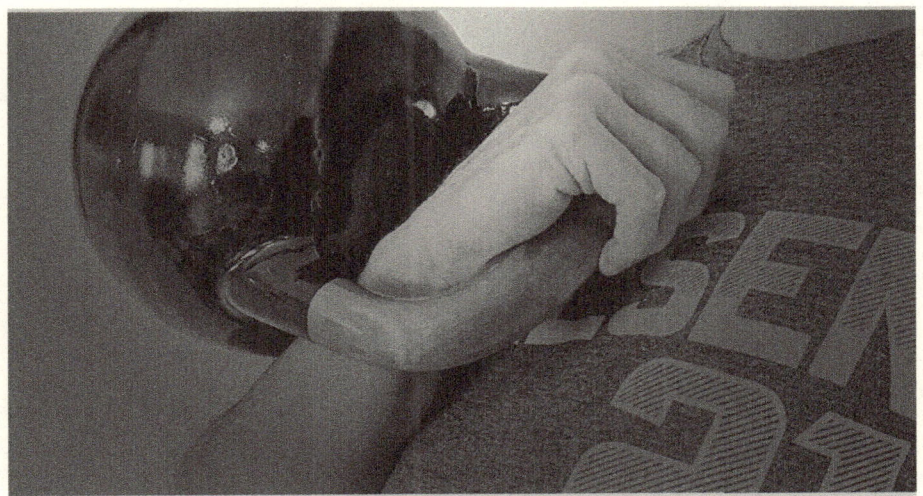

RACKING SAFETY GRIP

With this grip, the thumb is over the index finger, which are placed over the horn, and the remaining fingers are tucked behind the handle. This grip is used when working with two Kettlebells to protect the fingers from getting caught between the two Kettlebell handles.

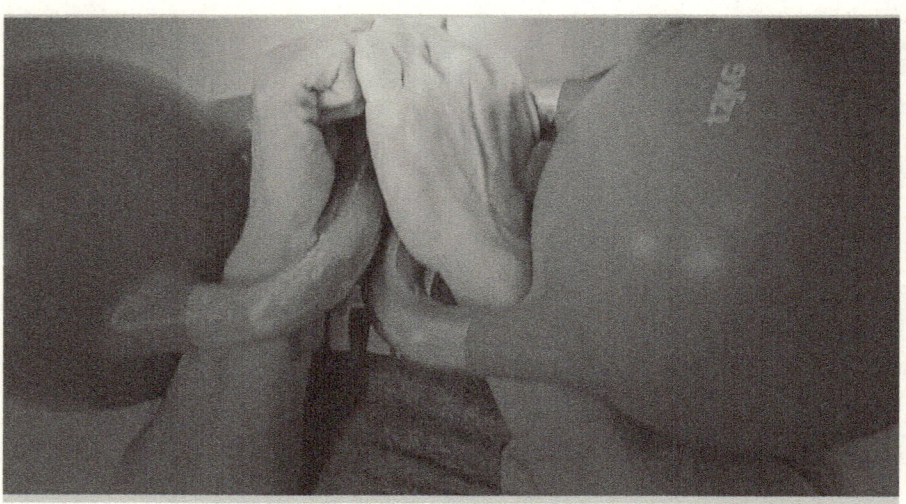

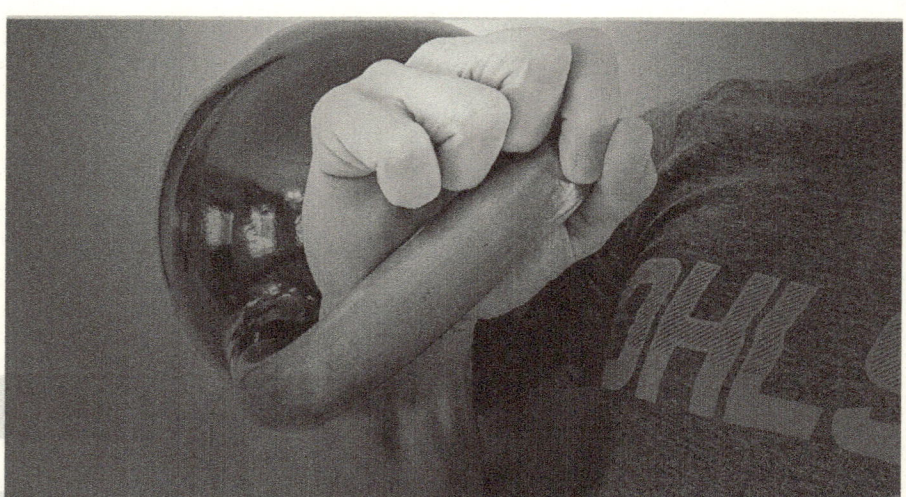

FLAT HAND GRIP

The hand is flat or straight, with all fingers pointing up and the thumb is around the horn. Can be employed for safety with two kettlebells, racking, or in overhead lock-out.

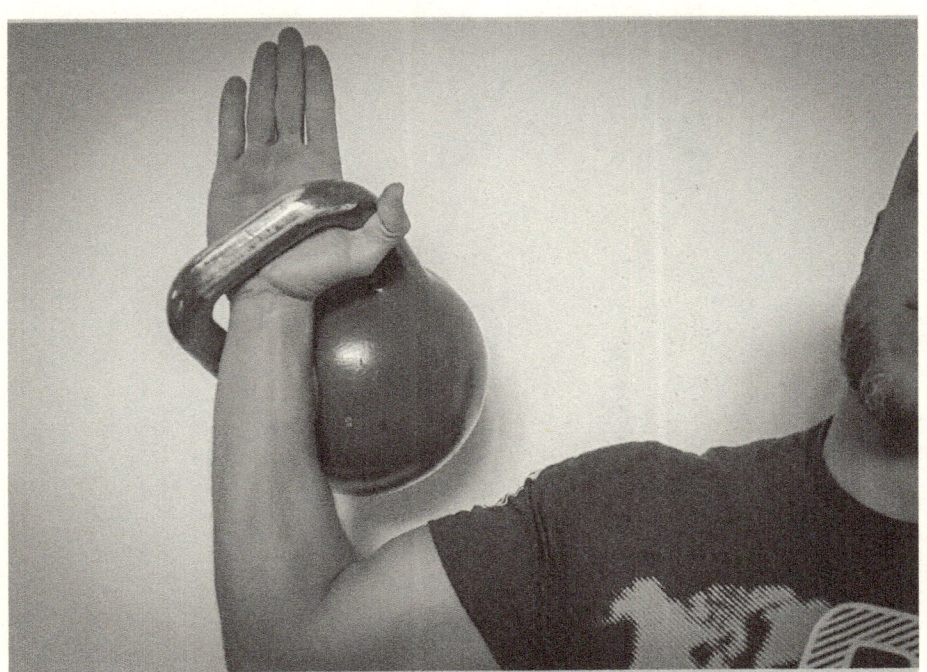

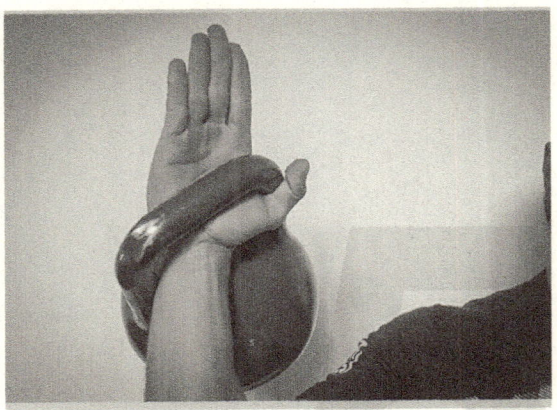

PINCH GRIP

With this grip, the thumb and fingers are used to pick up the Kettlebell by the base of the kettlebell; this can be performed only with a smaller classic Kettlebell. Used for working grip strength.

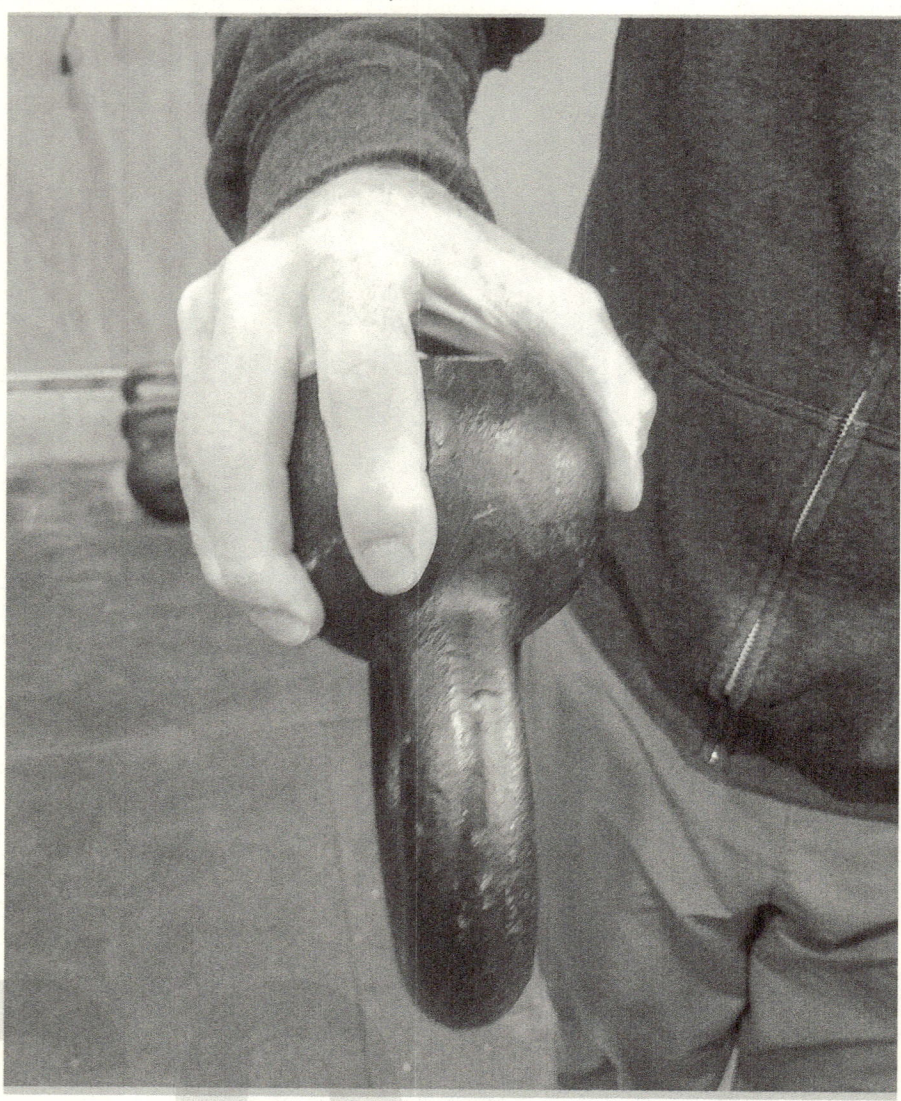

Photo provided by Robert Gagnon SFG II
www.RobGagnon.com

FARMER GRIP

Grip: middle of the handle.

Handle: one hand, four fingers and thumb locking the index finger down, or both the index and middle finger

Ideal for: farmer walks, suitcase dead lifts

With this grip the hand is placed in the middle of the handle, and used when carrying a heavy Kettlebell beside the body with farmer walks or dead lifts. It should be noted that although the farmer walk grip is usually with a firm grip — contrary to most other grips — you can perform farmer walks with a hook grip as well to challenge the fingers more.

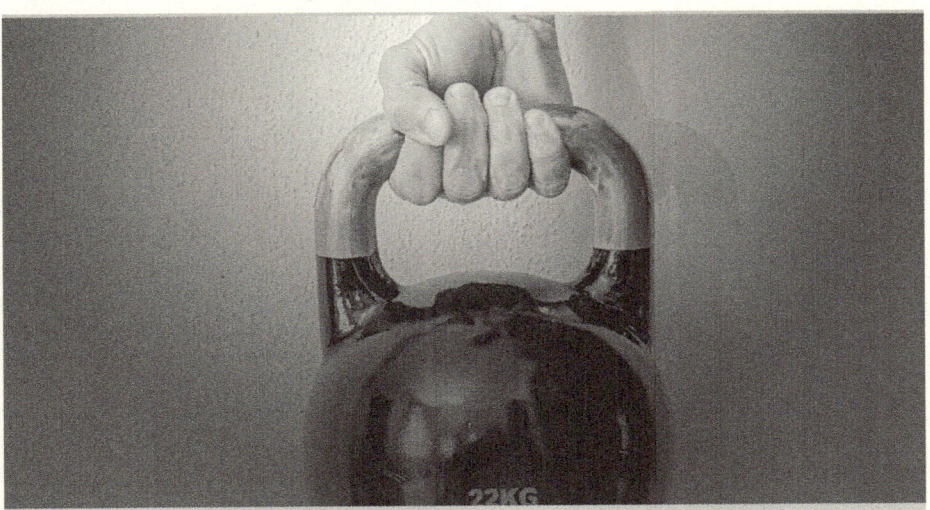

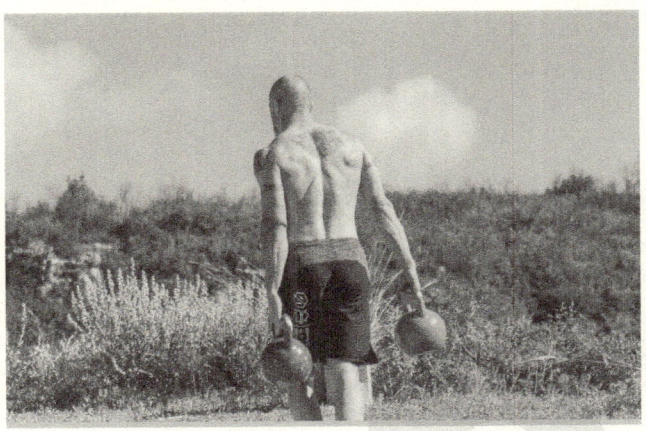

Farmer walks near Barranco Blanco on the Costa del Sol

BOTTOMS UP GRIP

Handle: one hand, four fingers and thumb crushing the handle

Ideal for: bottoms up press, bottoms up squat

This grip is performed with a strong and firm grip on the handle while the kettlebell is upside down, and used for bottoms up press or bottoms up Turkish get-up. The bottoms up grip is great to work on grip strength and stability.

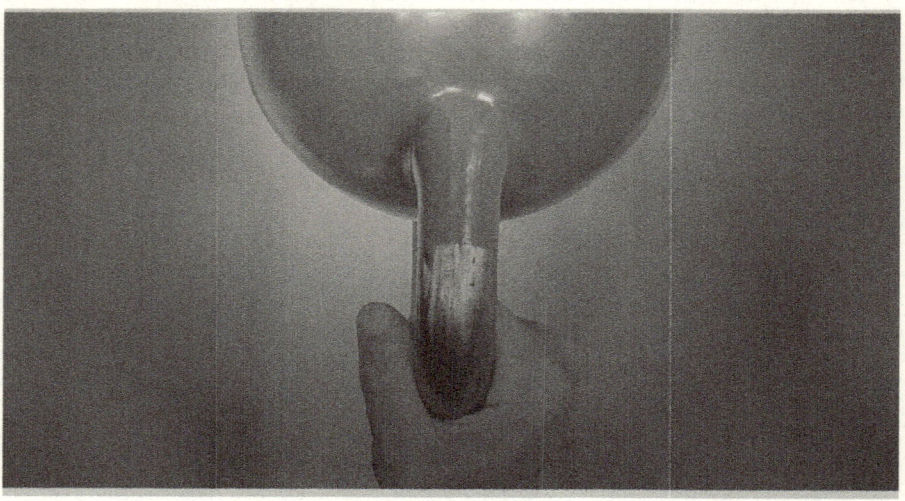

Make sure you check out our ebook Master The Kettlebell Press, which covers all kettlebell presses and is written by yours truly and Joe Daniels. http://bit.ly/2fN-V7d1

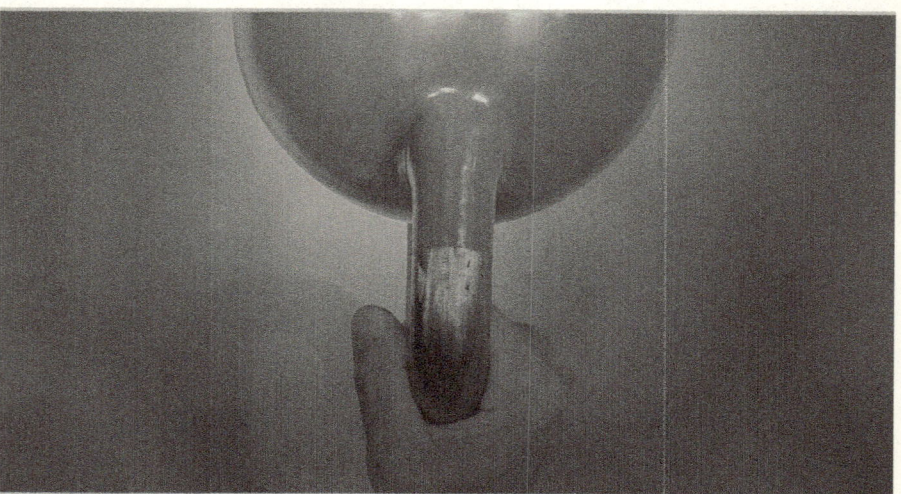

HORN GRIP

Handle: two hands, four fingers and thumb locking the index finger down on the horns

Ideal for: curls, lunge and twist, halo's

This grip is performed with both hands holding the horns, and is used for doing halos and bicep curls.

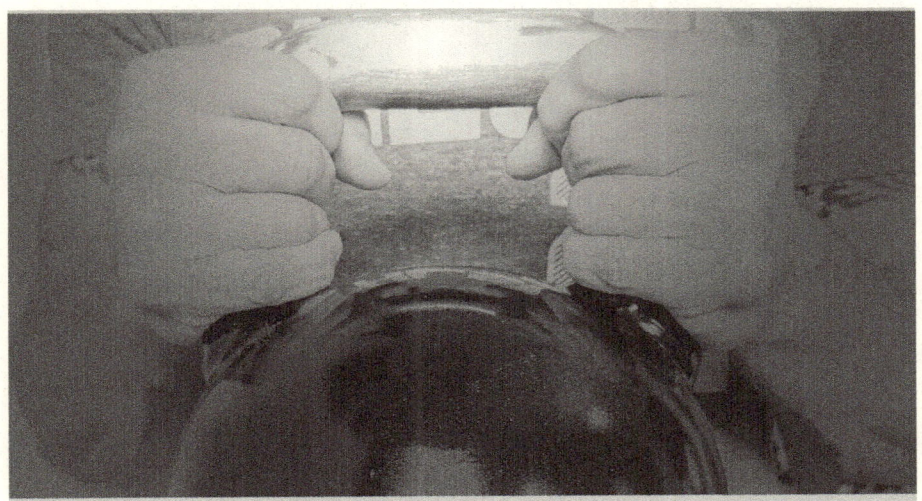

HORN GRIP UPSIDE DOWN

Handle: two hands, four fingers and thumb locking the index finger down on the horns

Ideal for: Russian twists, pull overs, halo's

This grip is performed with the hands holding the horns while the kettlebell is upside down, and can be used for pull overs and Russian twists.

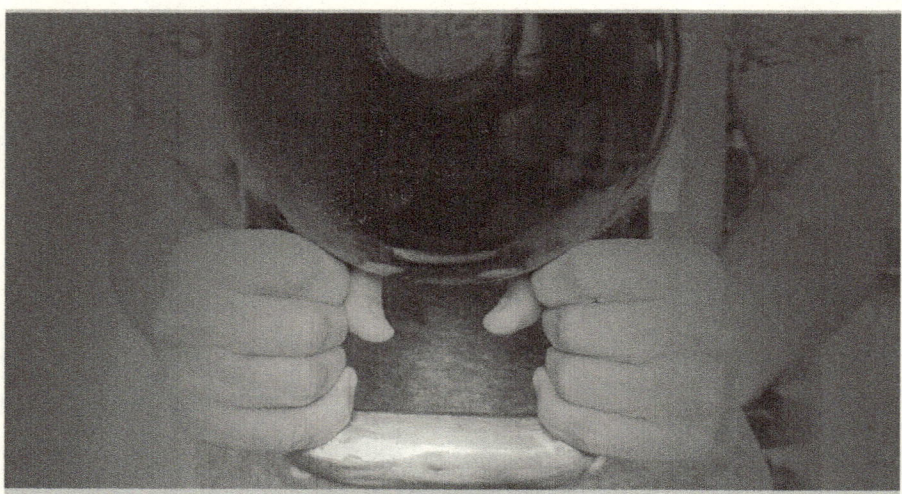

This is also a great grip to work on wrist strength with lateral wrist movement. You can do this in the air with a light bell, or have the handle resting on the ground with a heavier bell. When resting the handle on the ground and base is up, the objective is to slowly move the bell forward to where it almost touches the ground, slowly and controlled bringing it back towards you as far as possible.

If you do this drill in the air, it also works your biceps as you need to hold the forearms just above horizontal in a static position while moving the wrists. Of course this will also require you to activate your lats, chest, back, and abdominal muscles to provide a solid base from where to perform this drill.

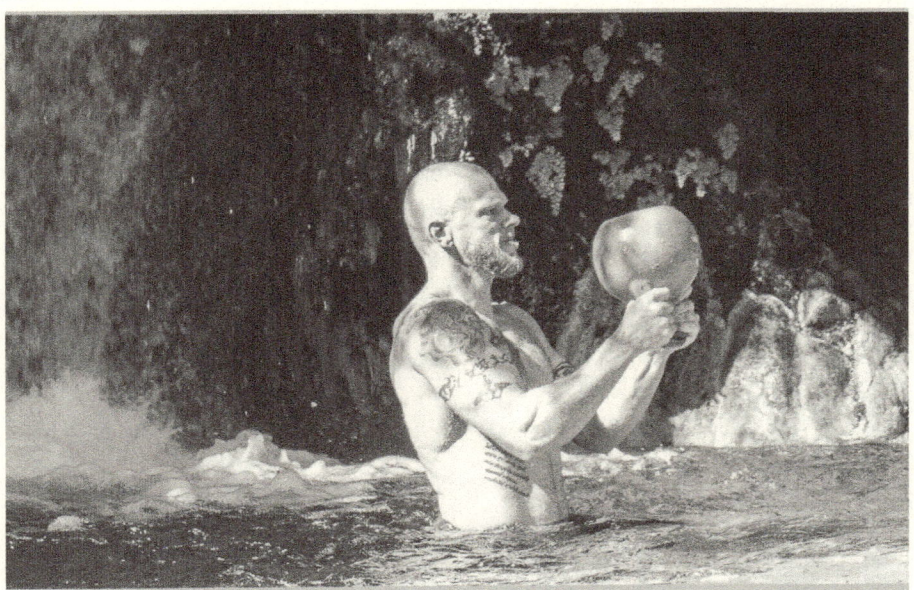

Taco Fleur in Barranco Blanco, Coin, Spain

Check out this video featuring the horn upside down grip in which I demonstrate the Russian twist and Caveman twist https://www.youtube.com/watch?v=_KbZ-no3KZdY

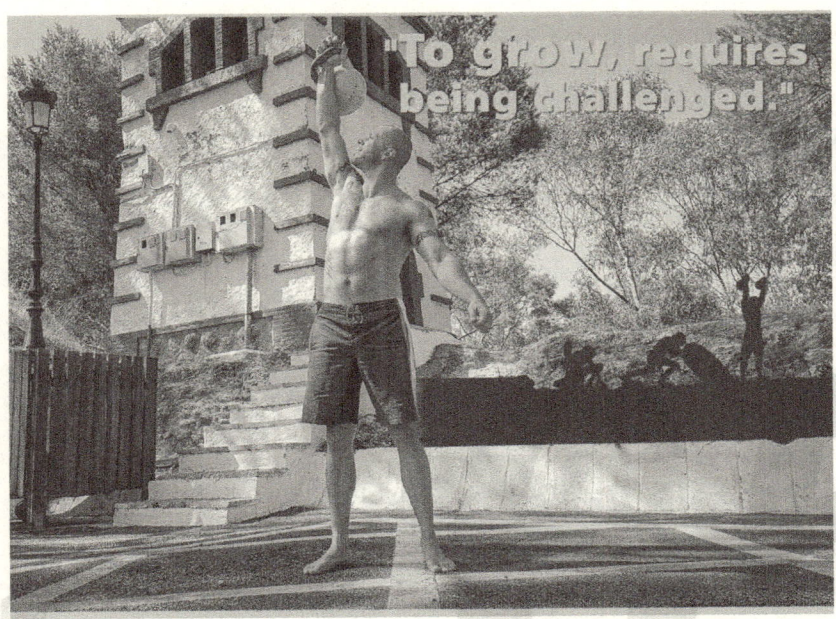

"To grow, requires being challenged."

CORNER GRIP

Handle: one hand, four fingers and thumb loose or locking the index finger down

Ideal for: around the body, figure eight

This grip is performed with the hand holding the handle in the corner, i.e. where the handle and horn intersects, used for around the body and figure eights. A corner grip is mostly employed for passing the kettlebell to the other hand, whether you're juggling or switching arms.

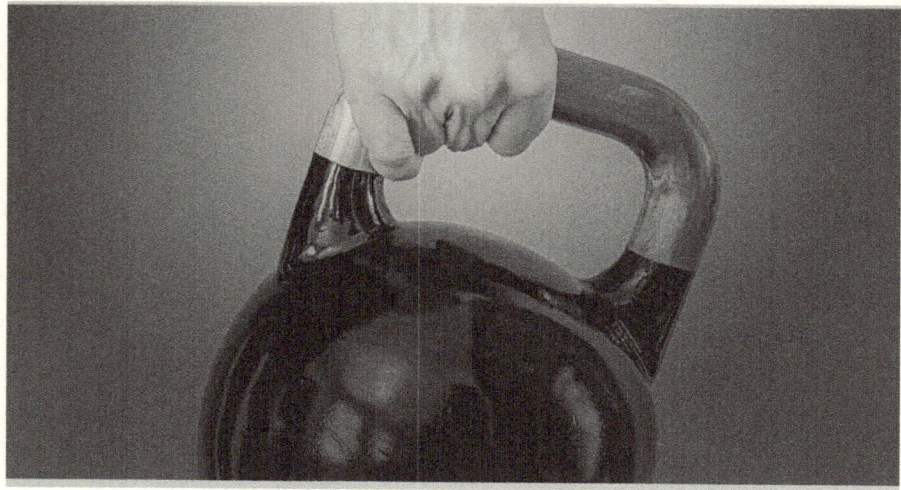

Corner grips with or without a finger lock like demonstrated in the following photo can also be used for single arm swings and snatches. Having your hand positioned there means it's already where it needs to end up in overhead position.

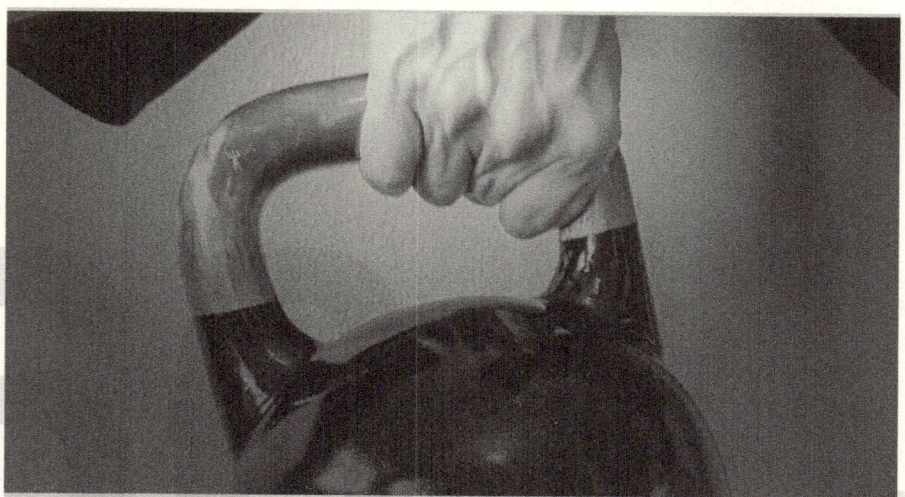

OPEN HAND HORN GRIP

Handle: two hands, all fingers slightly squeezing the bell and the thumbs folded around the bottom of the horns

Ideal for: laying down chest presses, front squats, skull crushers

With this grip both hands are used, palms are open and slightly squeezing the bell, which is resting within the palms; the thumbs are folded around the bottom of the horns. This grip is used for front squats and skull crushers.

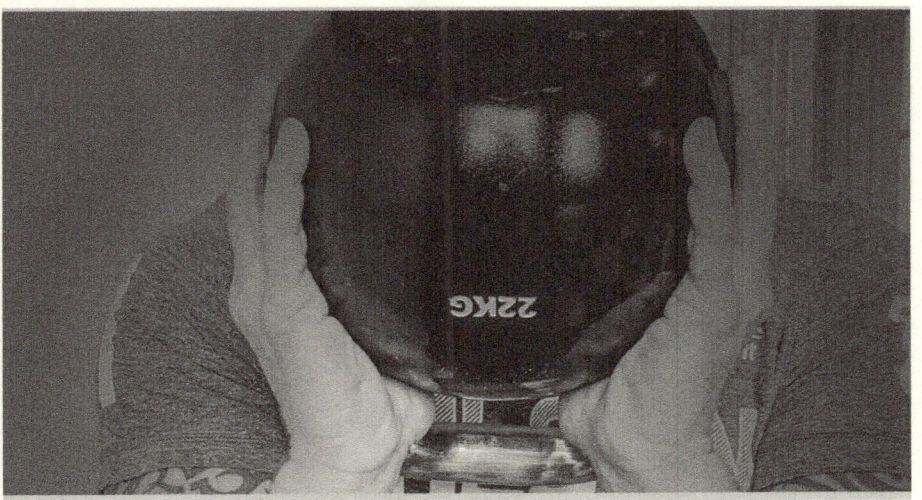

LOOSE GRIP

Handle: one hand, four fingers and thumb loosely around the handle

Ideal for: any press variation, any overhead work, racking

This grip is performed by keeping your fingers loose rather than tightly closed and squeezing, and is used for the overhead position in presses and snatches.

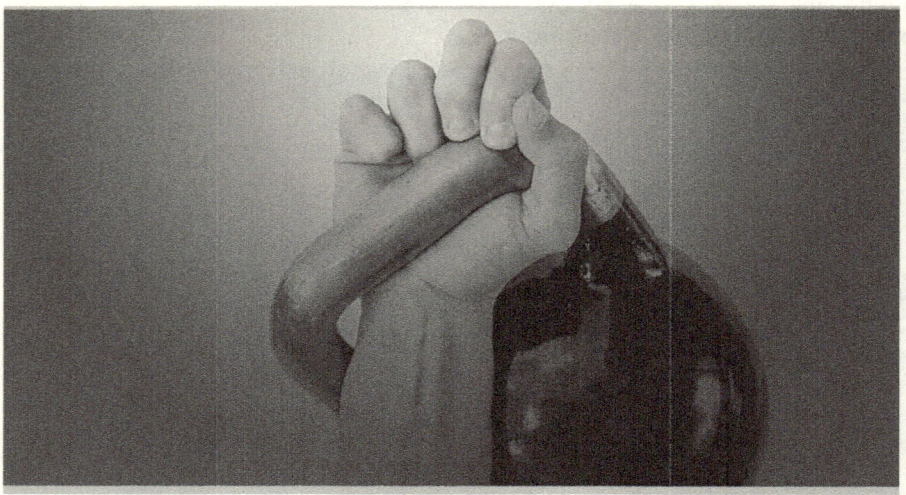

A great analogy to get the idea across for CrossFitters is thinking about a false grip.

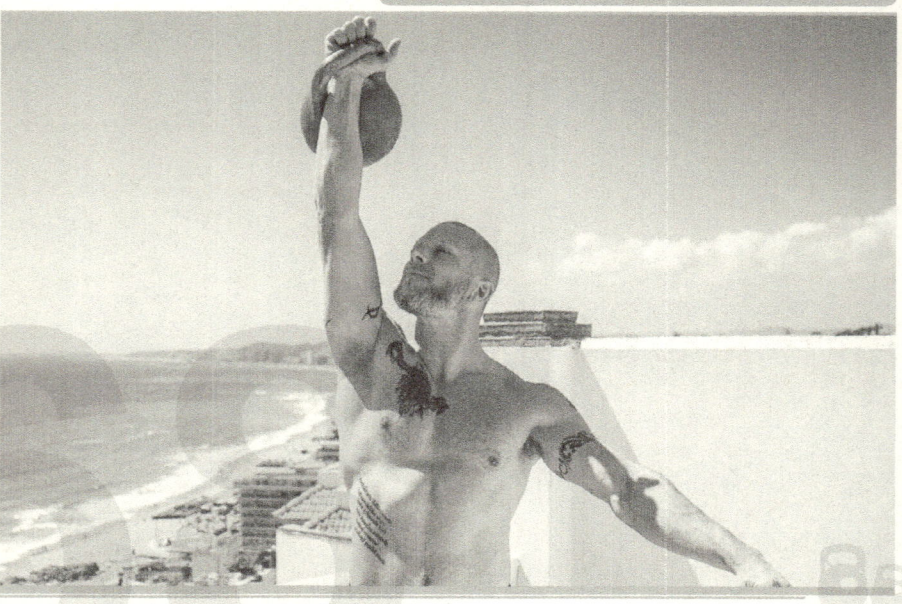

INTERLOCKING GRIP

Handle: two hands, all fingers interlocking and thumb through the corners

Ideal for: racking rest, anything performed with a rack, front squats

This grip is performed by interlocking the fingers of both hands, elbows tight into the side of the body, and is used for front squats or racked lunges.

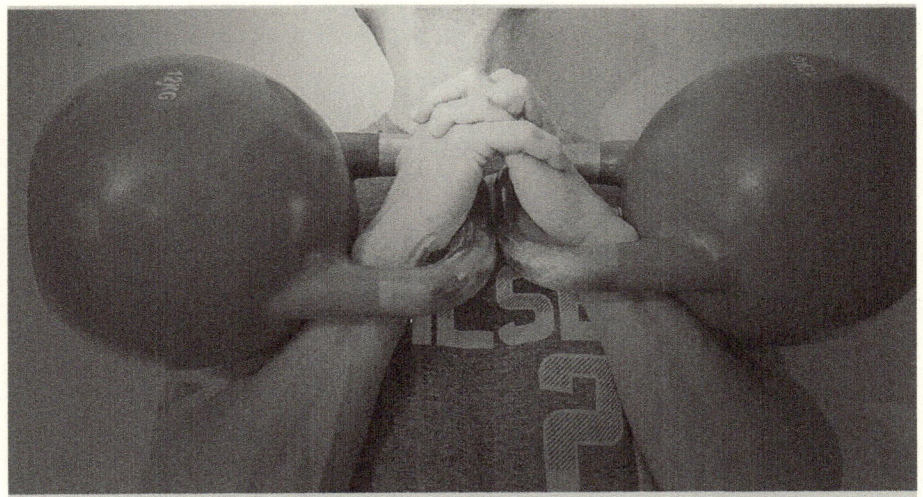

STACKING GRIP

Handle: two hands, several fingers holding on to the handle of the stacked kettlebell

Ideal for: racking rest, anything going rack to overhead

This grip is performed by placing the handles on top of each other and several fingers holding on to the second handle while the top hand is over the bottom hand; used for resting or anything going overhead like press, push press, or jerk.

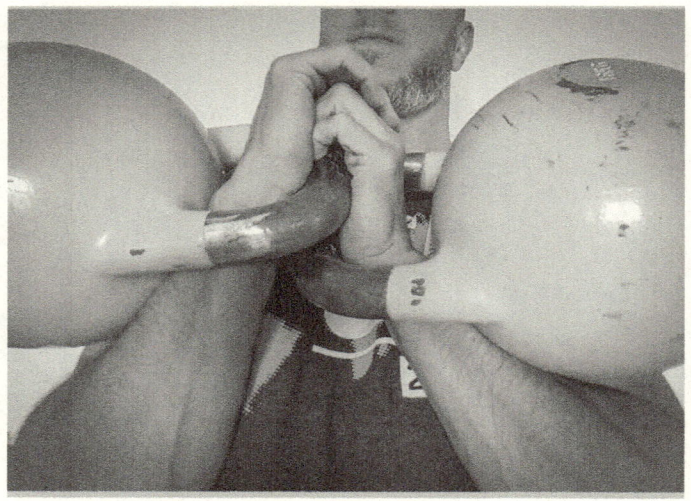

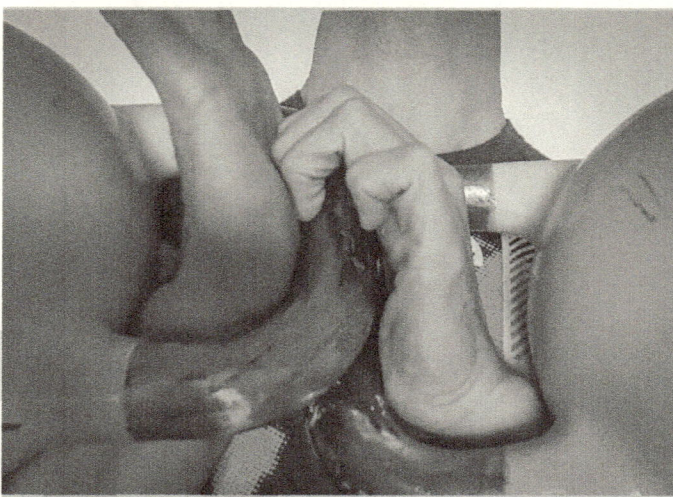

The bottom hand and the area the fingers grip on the top handle

OPEN PALM GRIP

Handle: handle is resting against the underside of the forearm

Ideal for: increasing difficulty of presses

This grip is performed with the bell resting in the open palm, and handle against the underside of the forearm. Great for working on wrist strength.

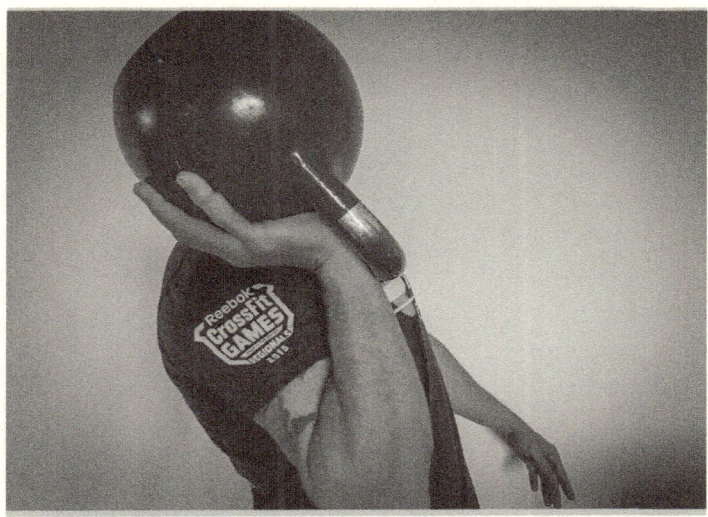

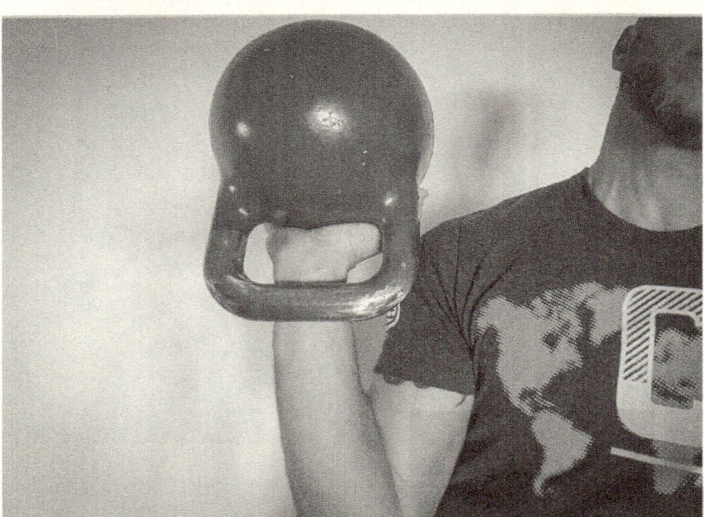

Watch a video where I employ the open palm grip https://www.youtube.com/watch?v=ZtnLJl9m1gU

WAITERS GRIP

Handle: the handle does not come into play

Ideal for: increasing difficulty of presses

This grip is performed with the base resting on the open palm. Great for working on wrist strength. This grip is named for obvious reasons; the way the kettlebell rests on the palm resembles that of a waiter carrying a tray.

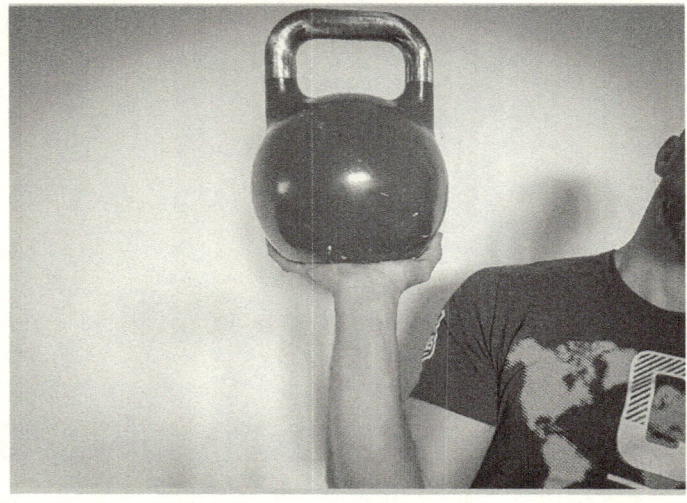

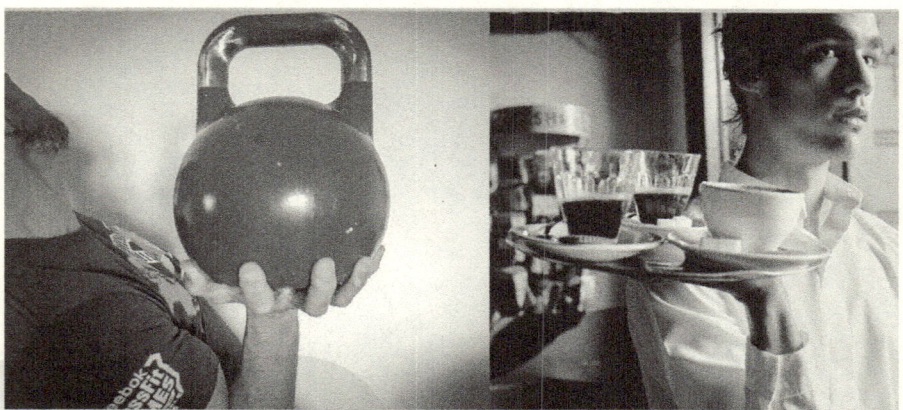

Watch a video where I employ the waiters grip https://www.youtube.com/watch?v=YwF27hFHSEo

Once you get into kettlebell juggling, you can swing and catch the kettlebell directly into waiters grip; from there you can perform an overhead squat. This variation requires a more explosive swing to get the kettlebell high and flip into waiters grip.

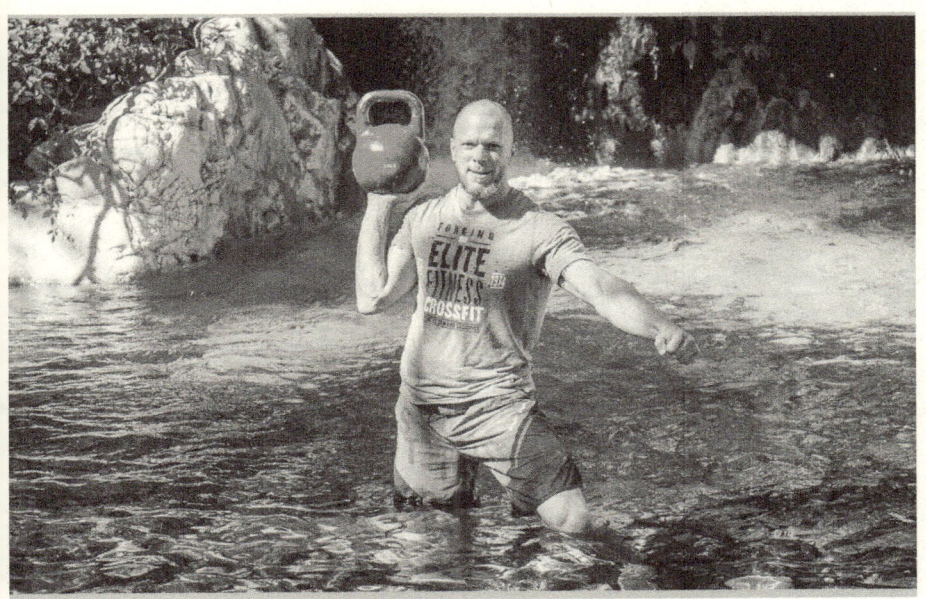

GOBLET GRIP

Handle: the handle does not come into play

Ideal for: front-squat

This grip is performed with the palms pressing around the bell; handle is up or down. The grip is named for obvious reasons; the shape of the kettlebell with handle down resembles that of a goblet. With the handle facing up, this grip is called Reverse Goblet Grip. The higher you go up the bell with your palms, the harder you need to squeeze, palms towards the bottom, and the bell is resting more within the palms.

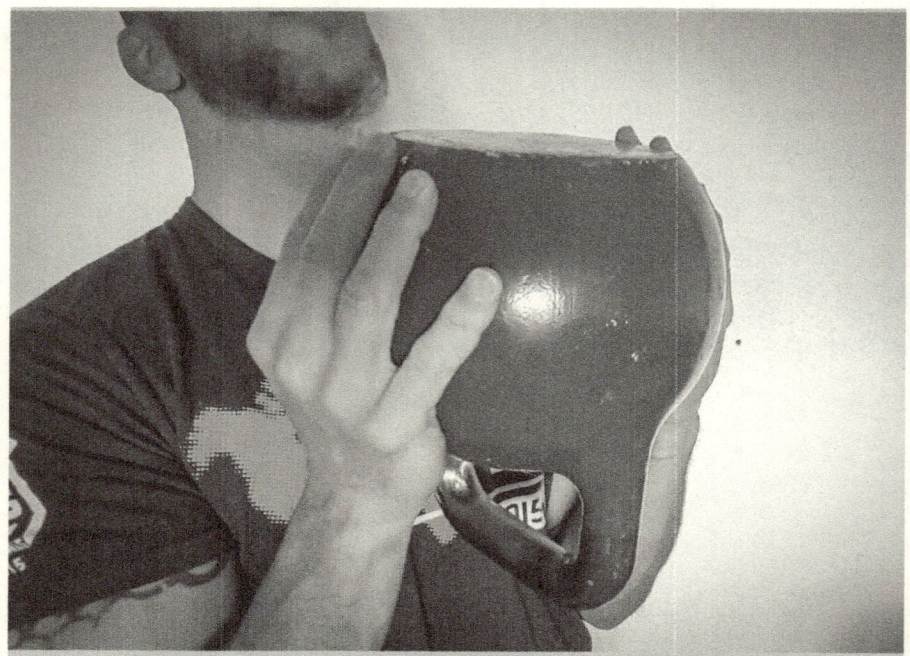

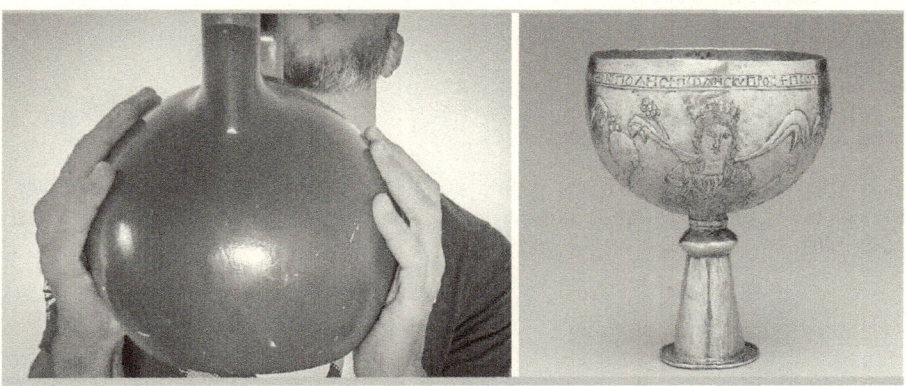

The reverse goblet grip and a golden goblet

There is a lot of confusion about the Goblet Grip, and for that reason I wrote an article which I recommend reading. www.cavemantraining.com/caveman-kettle-bells/goblet-squat-rather-goblet-grip/

You can watch a video demonstrating the Goblet Grip in a Goblet Squat. www.youtube.com/watch?v=peuGSnbgXEk

CRUSH GRIP

Handle: the handle does not come into play

Ideal for: front-squat, static hold

This grip is performed with the palms crushing the bell; handle is up or down. Similar to the goblet grip, but more crushing with the palms. Great for working the pectoralis.

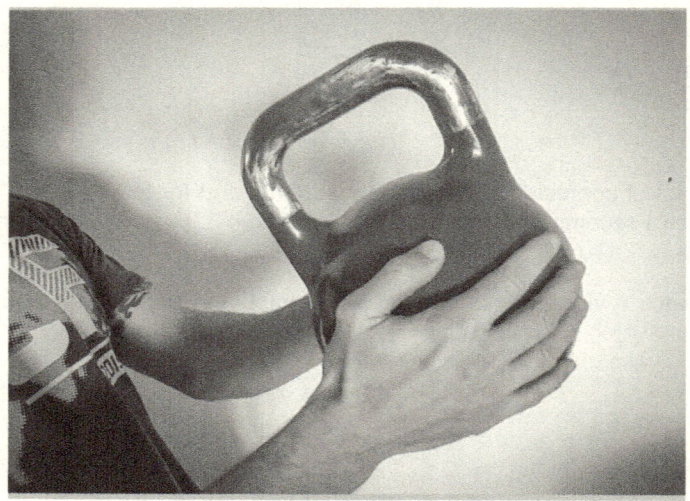

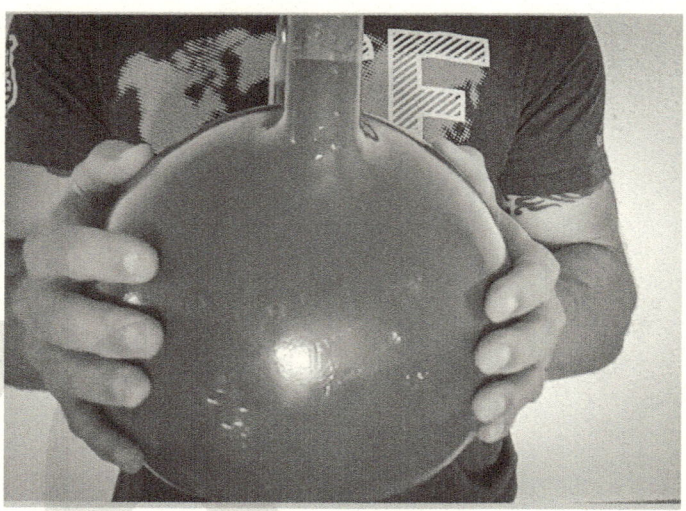

THUMB GRIP (AKA NOOB GRIP)

Handle: The handle is resting more on the heel of the thumb than with the loose grip.

Ideal for: press, front-squat

The bell rests on the inside of the arm, complete opposite of the loose grip; the handle is resting more on the heel of the thumb. Great for shifting the weight from the outside of the arm to the inside. Full range reps from racking are not possible with this grip. Try this one with the side press starting above the shoulder and returning above the shoulder.

I like to call this the noob grip, as this is the grip a lot of new people use the first ever time they lift a kettlebell without instruction.

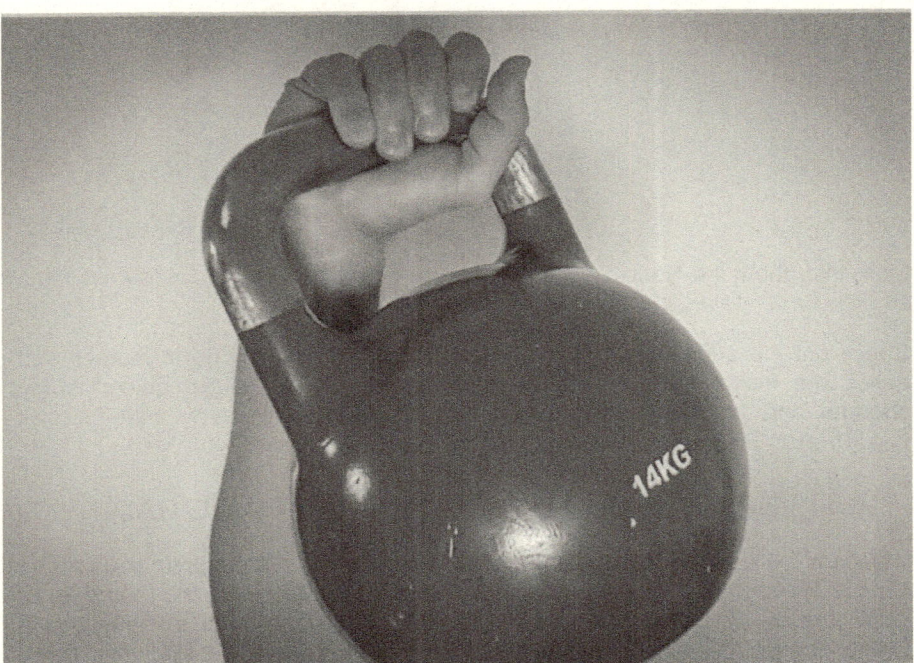

Find out why I named this the Noob Grip and why it's such a great grip to employ after you learned all other grips. www.cavemantraining.com/caveman-kettlebells/24-unconventional-kettlebell-exercises-three-broken/

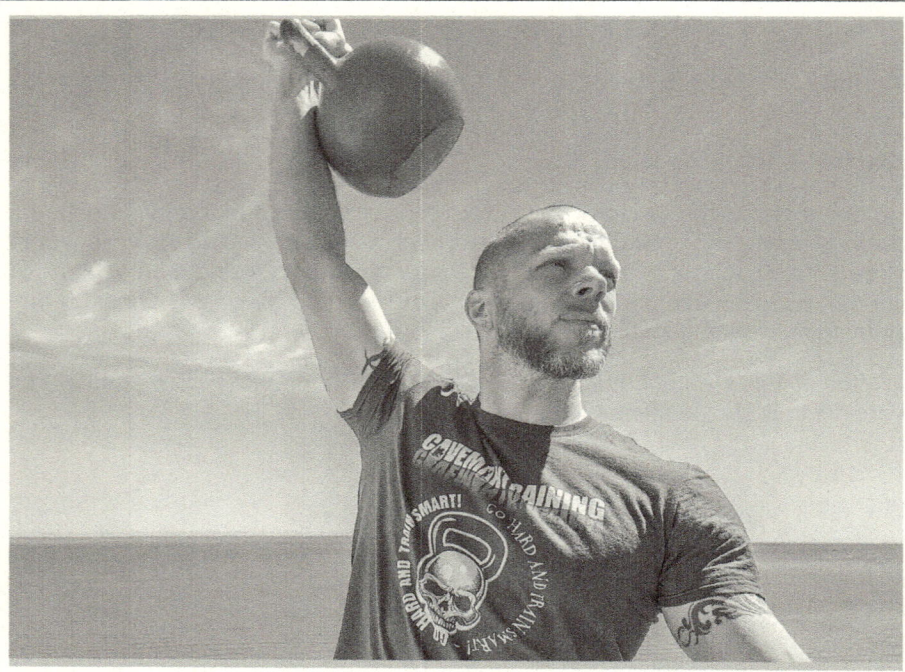

Noob grip press

More info about the Noob Grip Squat can be found here: www.cavemantraining.com/caveman-kettlebells/even-kettlebell-squat-bro/

Check out the combination of Noob Grip Squat and Press. Try it yourself and notice the instability it provides, which is great once you've gained some strength and technique by implementing common grips. www.youtube.com/watch?v=Q8t05MbK_R4

THUMB UP OR THUMB DOWN? PERFORMANCE GAIN?

Does it really matter? Yes it does. It sounds like something trivial and insignificant to discuss which way the thumb should be pointing during the swing, clean, or snatch… who cares which way they're pointing, right?

If you're swinging a kettlebell one-handed you can change the direction your thumb is pointing (forearm supination/pronation); you can go through the legs with the thumb up or down; even anything in between up or down is fine, like sideways pointing medially. In fact, if you're going for endurance swings, you might want to consider thumb up, which requires less tricep activation.

Whether your thumb is pointing up, inward, or down is also a matter of personal preference. Try a different version and see what works best for you; however, one thing is for sure: At the top of the swing, your thumb should not be pointing down, which means your elbow is pointing up. Keeping your arm extended in this position becomes much harder.

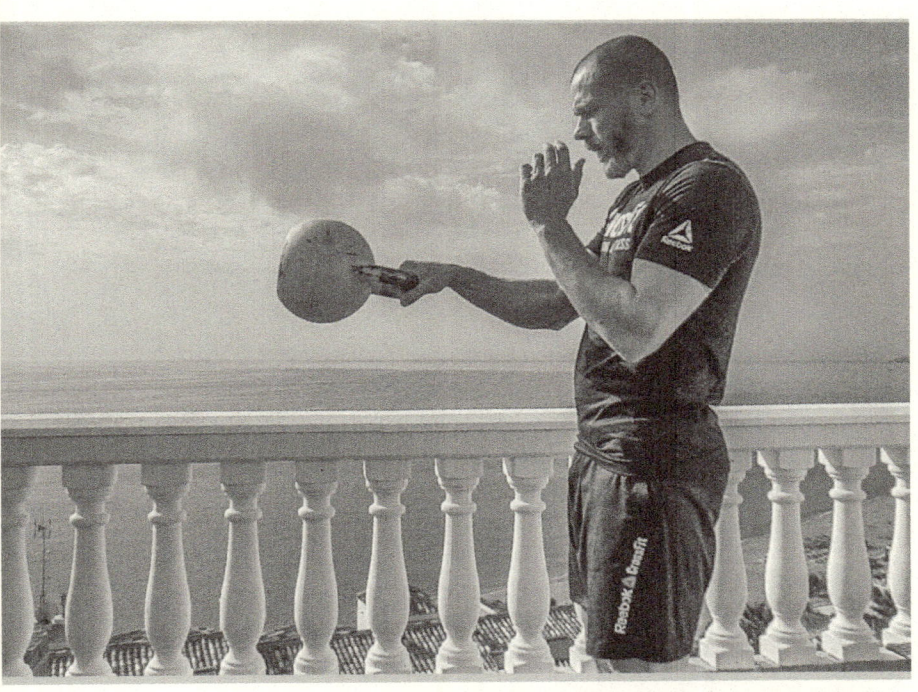

Thumb pointing medially, during swing.

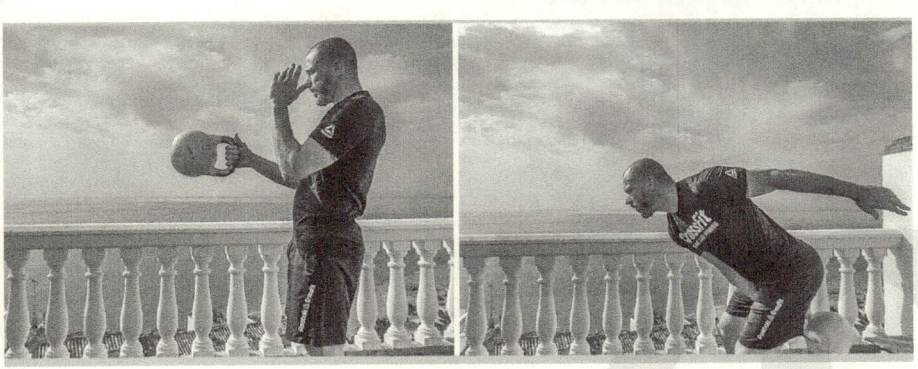

Thumb pointing up, during up, and back swing.

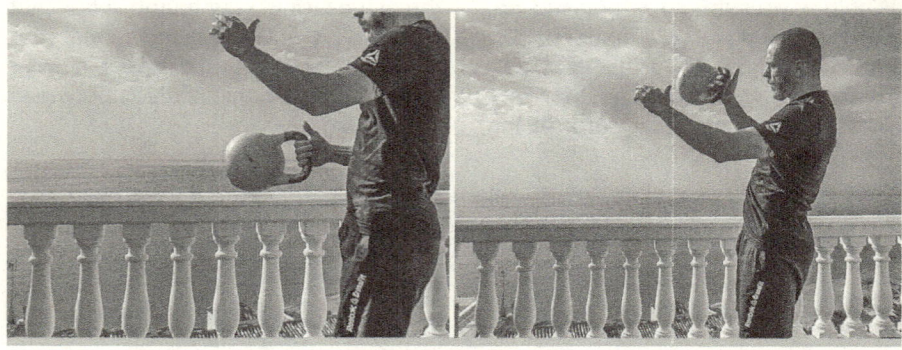

Thumb pointing up, during the clean, and snatch.

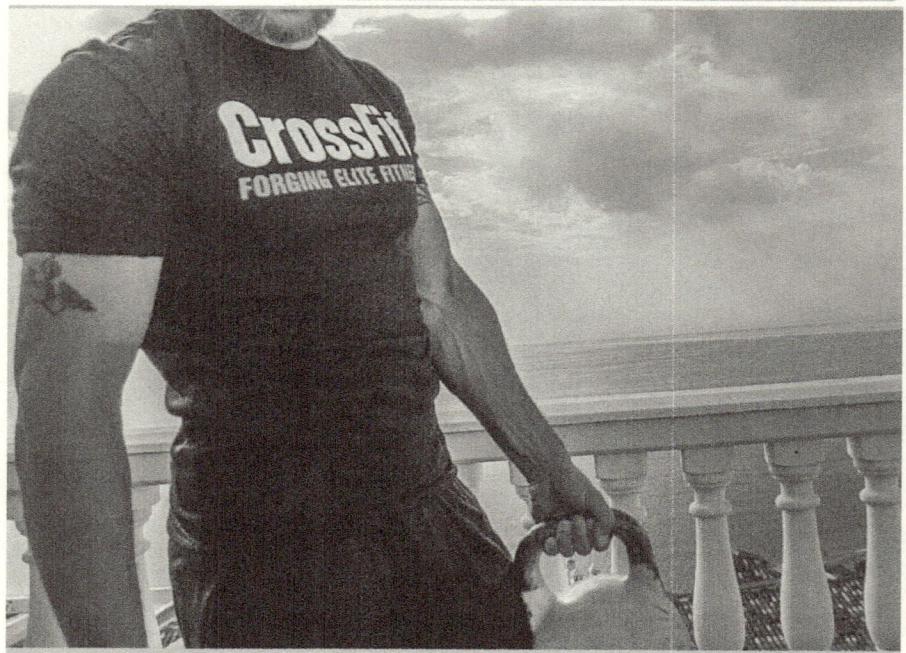

Thumb up.

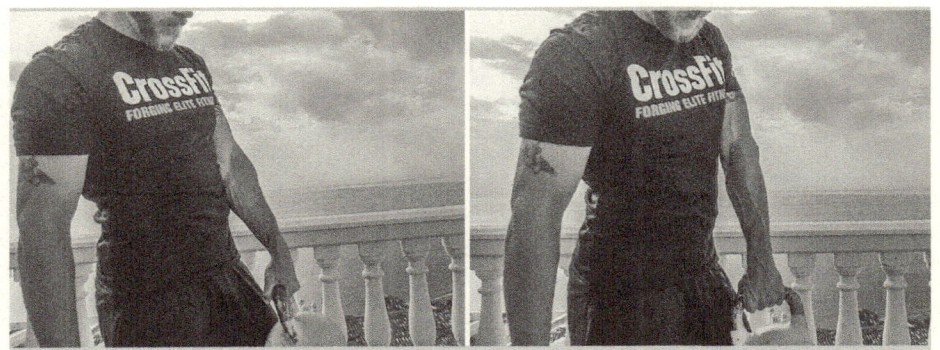

Thumb medially, and down.

Thumb should never be pointing down on the upward phase of the swing.

I learned the following from Steve Cotter in a certification course: Steve explained the concept of the thumb up and letting the triceps rest on the ribs. This works really well when you're doing a fluid style of swing; your arm stays easily extended and supported by the torso until it disconnects through generated force.

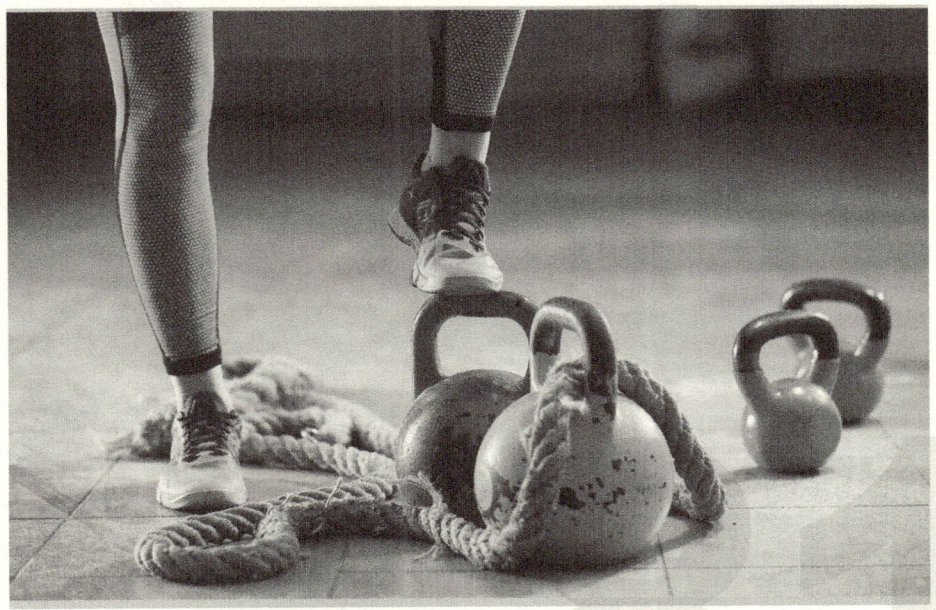

BASIC DOUBLE ARM SWING INSTRUCTIONS

The Kettlebell Swing is the foundation for many other kettlebell exercises; therefore, it is important you become proficient in this exercise and understand the finer details.

The kettlebell swing is a full body exercise and really helps to strengthen the posterior chain muscles. The posterior chain muscles are comprised of many muscles, but some of the main muscles are biceps femoris, gluteus maximus, erector spinae muscle group, trapezius, and posterior deltoids.

The kettlebell swing movement pattern is very similar to the conventional deadlift; the main difference is that the weight swings, and the movement is explosive. The hinge movement of the hips is the same. When referring to the kettlebell swing, in most cases that means the Russian swing; the other popular (but different) swing is the American swing.

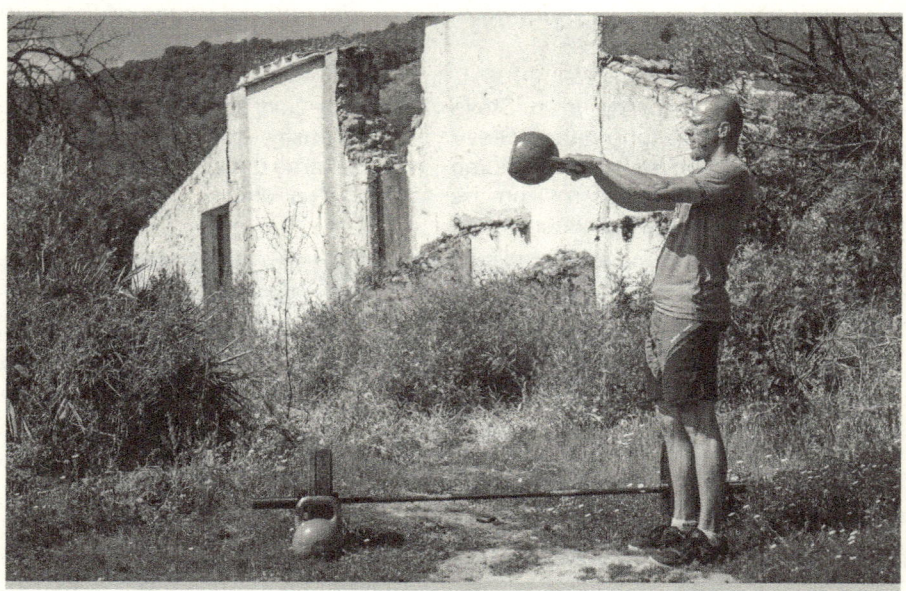

Double-arm swing AKA Russian swing

To perform the kettlebell swing:
- Stand in spine-neutral position with feet slightly wider than shoulder-width apart with the kettlebell in-front of you
- Maintain a neutral spine with core braced at all times during the swing
- Keep the feet flat on the ground at all times to be able to push into the ground and activate the hamstring muscles to pull the pelvis and propel the bell forward

- Keep the arms straight at all times (this can change once you've mastered the swing, but that's for another book; for now keep the arms straight)
- Leave the arms relaxed and only use them only as a pendulum, so the kettlebell can swing back and forth freely
- Hold the kettlebell by the handle with both hands and a loose grip
- Pull the kettlebell off the ground and through the legs
- The height of the kettlebell should be around knee height; see illustration of the hip hinge, only difference being the arms are coming through the legs
- Explosively bringing the hips forward
- The upper body follows and comes upright to propel the kettlebell forward
- Do not involve your shoulders to lift the kettlebell upward; let the power from the lower-body and the coming upright of the upper body propel the kettlebell
- Do not hyper extend the back when bringing the hips forward; in other words do not extend your back

Note: Proper hip extension is different and might be slightly required when working with extremely heavy weights to create proper weight distribution

- Make sure to squeeze the glutes to pull the pelvis up

- The top of the swing is when the kettlebell is motionless in the air for a split second

- The kettlebell usually reaches about chest height, but keep in mind that the kettlebell needs to swing only as high as the force generated by your lower-body will move it

- At the top of the swing remember:
    - Chest out and shoulders back (thoracic extension)
    - Engage the core
    - Squeeze the glutes
    - Legs are straight

- It's time to start thinking about breaking at the hips when the kettlebell starts to fall down

- Delay breaking of the hips as long as possible to prevent unbalanced movement

    The heavier the weight, the more fatigue is present, the longer the delay of breaking at the hips—more details in our dedicated kettlebell swing book

- The kettlebell should come through the legs approximately around the knees

- You should be able to put another kettlebell between your legs and not hit it

- Elbows/forearms should be making contact around the waist line, and part of the wrists around the upper thighs

- Exhale through the mouth on the up-phase

- Inhale through the nose on the down-phase

- Break at the hips and push them backwards (AKA hip hinge)

Try to keep the knees above the ankles as much as possible/shins vertical

- You should feel tension on the hamstrings when pushing the hips back, and remember that this version of the swing is not a squat

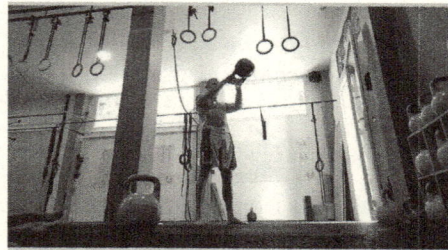
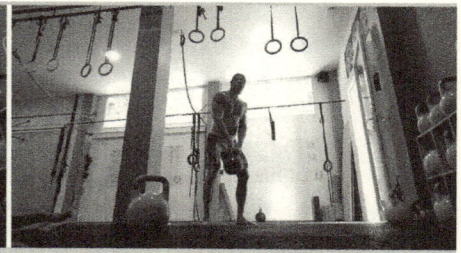

Delay of the hip hinge.

BAD FORM

✗   Pick a weight too light and you don't get the resistance needed to activate the right muscles

✗   Pick a weight too heavy, and your form will go out the door

✗   No hip drive – will fatigue quickly in shoulders and lower back

✗   Coming too low – lower back will start hurting

✗   Hyper extending the back – prone to more serious injury

✗   Happy feet – not able to activate the right muscles

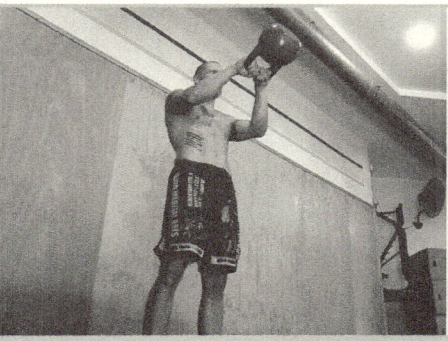
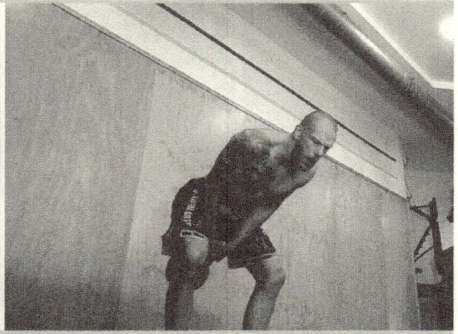

Remember, not every human being is built the same; therefore certain moves might not work the same for your body as for someone else. Always use common sense, and adjust the exercise as required while staying within the safety guidelines.

As long as the exercise is performed safely, any slight adjustments should be fine. If you are unsure, join our discussion group on Facebook and post your question. **And last but not least, there are hundreds of correct variations to swing a kettlebell.**

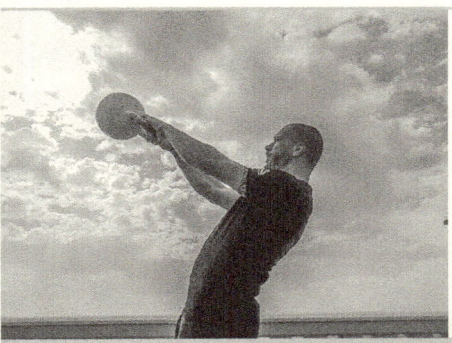
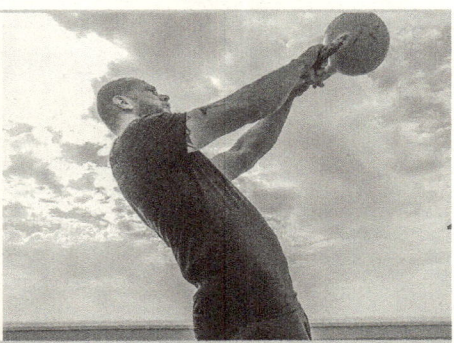

Excessive hyperextension of the back, lumbar in particular. Not good.

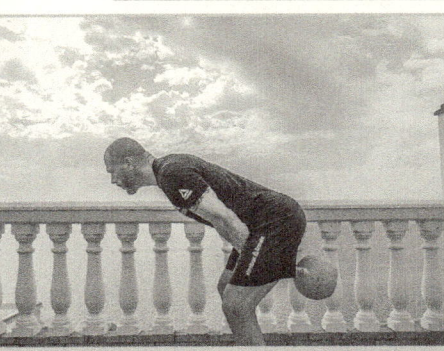
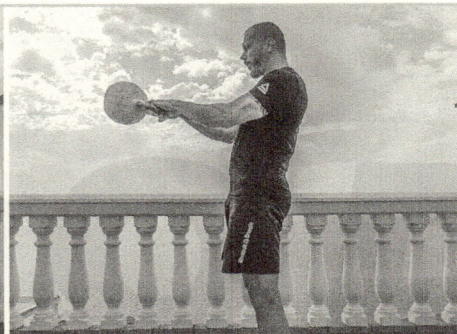

End of the back swing, and floating phase of the up swing.

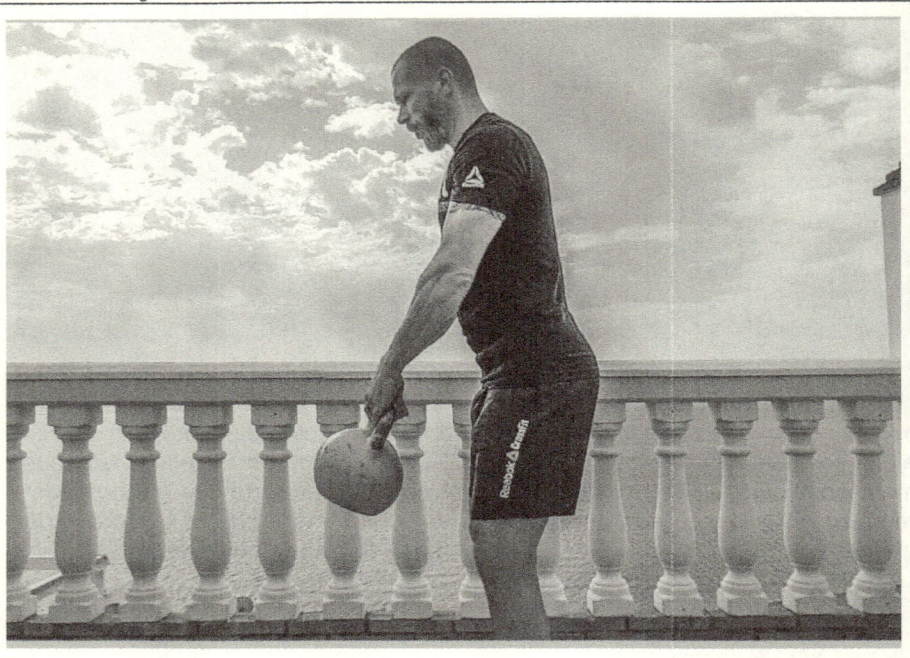
Hip hinge initiated.

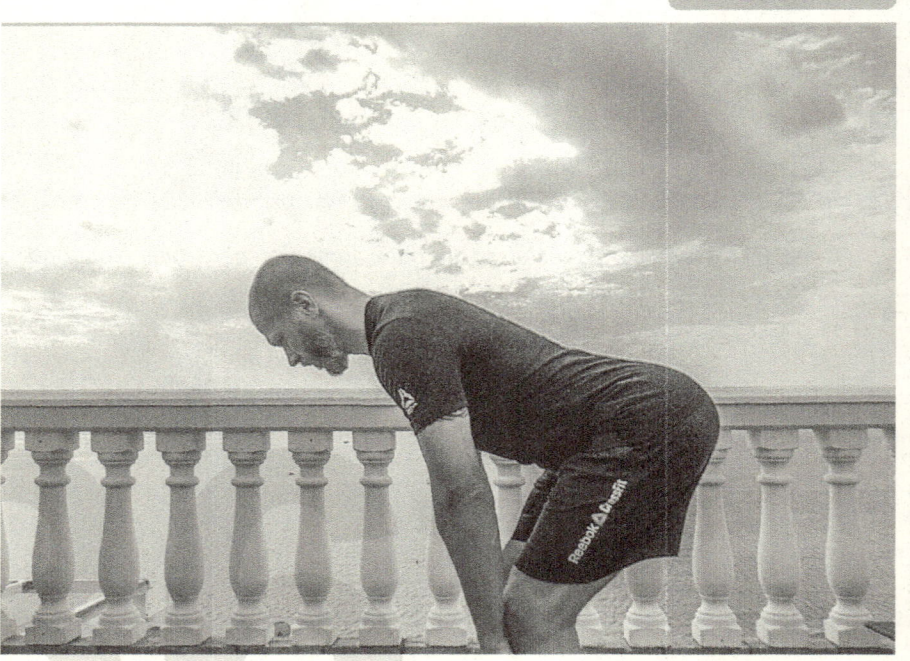
Hip hinge continued.

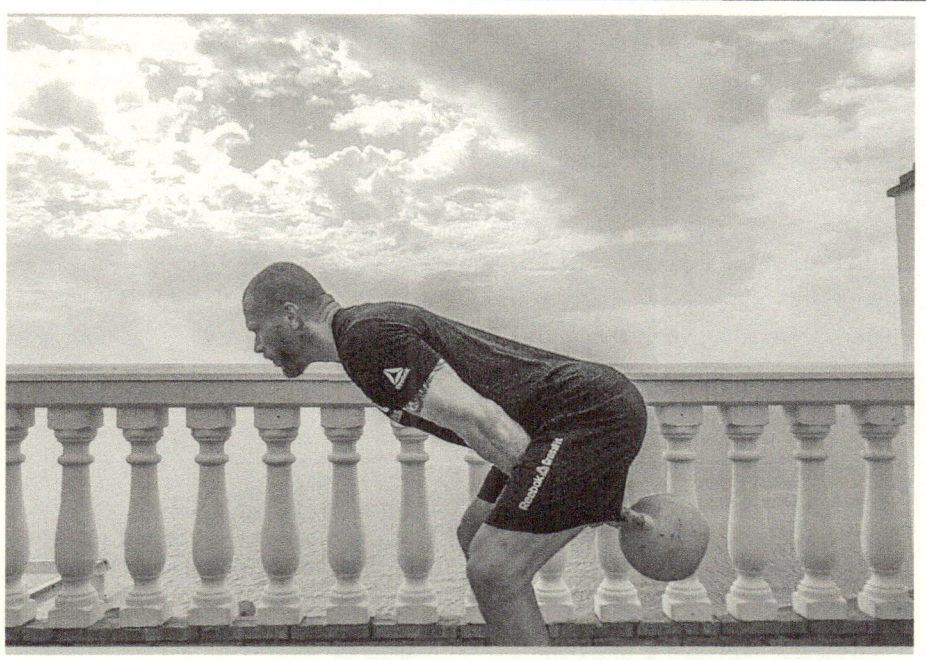

Insert performed. Direct the kettlebell toward the back.

Directing the kettlebell toward the back is what helps prevent bobbing of the kettlebell.

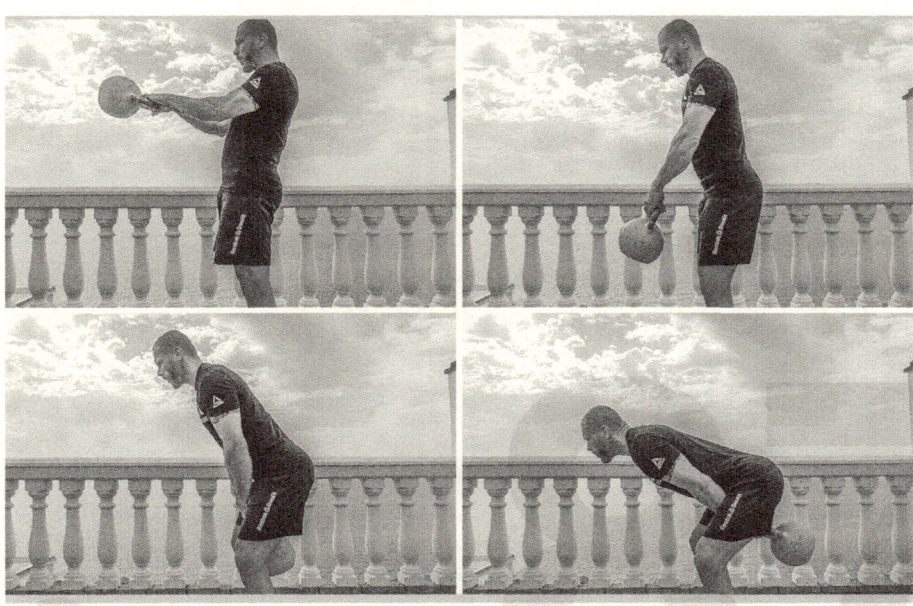

SQUAT AND HIP HINGE DEFINITION

Following is the definition of a squat and hip hinge; this is included so that you understand when something turns into a squat or when something is a hip hinge.

[Creative Commons License]

Definition of the squat:

Movement
- Torso remaining vertical as much as possible
- Hips always moving down

Hinge joints
- Hips, knees, and ankles

A squat is performed in standing position with the objective being to move the hip joints as close to the ground as possible. This is achieved through flexion in 3 joints: flexion in the hip joints, flexion in the knee joints, and dorsiflexion in the ankle joints.

If flexion is achieved in any of the joints that define the squat, but no maximum depth is achieved, then it's further defined by the approximate height; quarter squat; half squat; three-quarter squat; whereas maximum depth would be a full squat. A quick quarter squat can also be defined as a dip.

The objective of the squat exercise is to tax the quadriceps and gluteus maximus. A completely vertical position of the torso provides the maximum resistance for the quadriceps, and the more it moves towards horizontal, the more it removes resistance from the target muscles. Furthermore, a vertical position of the torso provides the most stable and safe spinal structure for the weighted squat. The torso should never break the angle of 45° flexion.

Definition of the hip hinge:

Movement
- Torso moving towards but never past horizontal
- Hips remaining at same height, or moving back and down

Hinge joints
- Fixed: hips
- Variable: knees

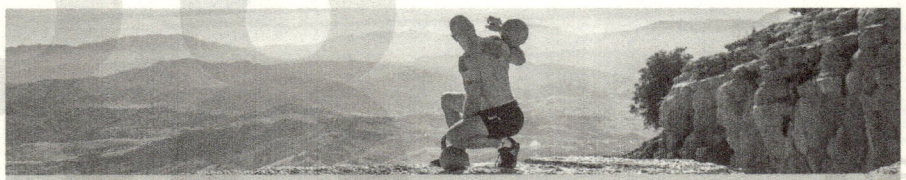

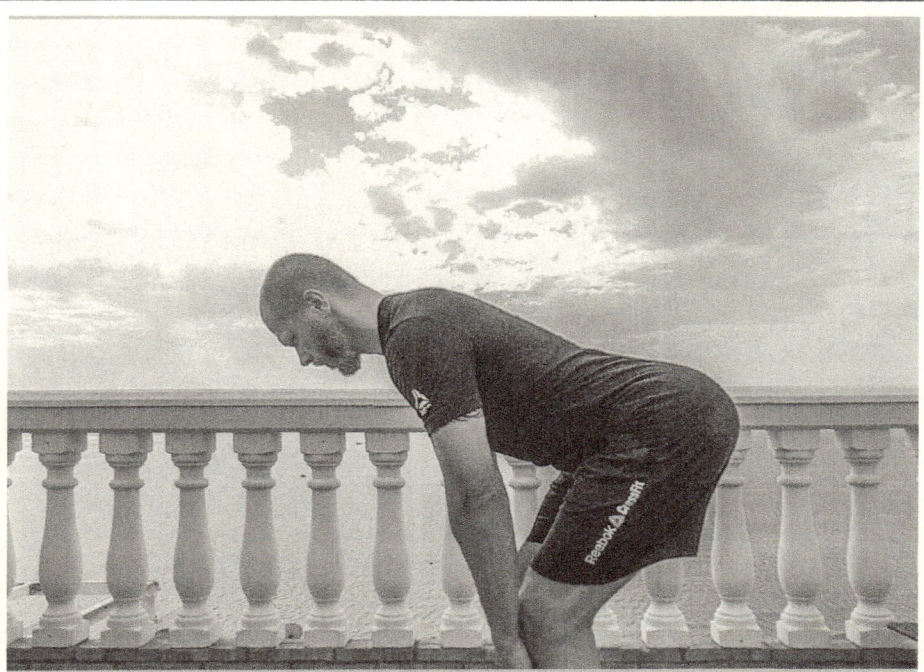

A hip hinge is performed in standing position, with the objective being to move the torso toward horizontal, this is achieved through flexion in the hip joints. The movement can also be accompanied by flexion in a second joint, that of the knees, which is cause for the hips to move down and backward. The function of added knee flexion is to create a more balanced weight distribution, especially with weighted hip hinges like deadlifts. If the ankle joints move and dorsiflexion is achieved, the definition of the movement changes to a squat.

The objective of the hip hinge exercise is to tax the gluteus maximus and hamstrings (hip extensors). A completely horizontal torso provides the maximum resistance for the hip flexors, and the more it moves towards vertical, the more resistance is removed.

The maximum recommended hip flexion is 45° for weighted hip hinges.

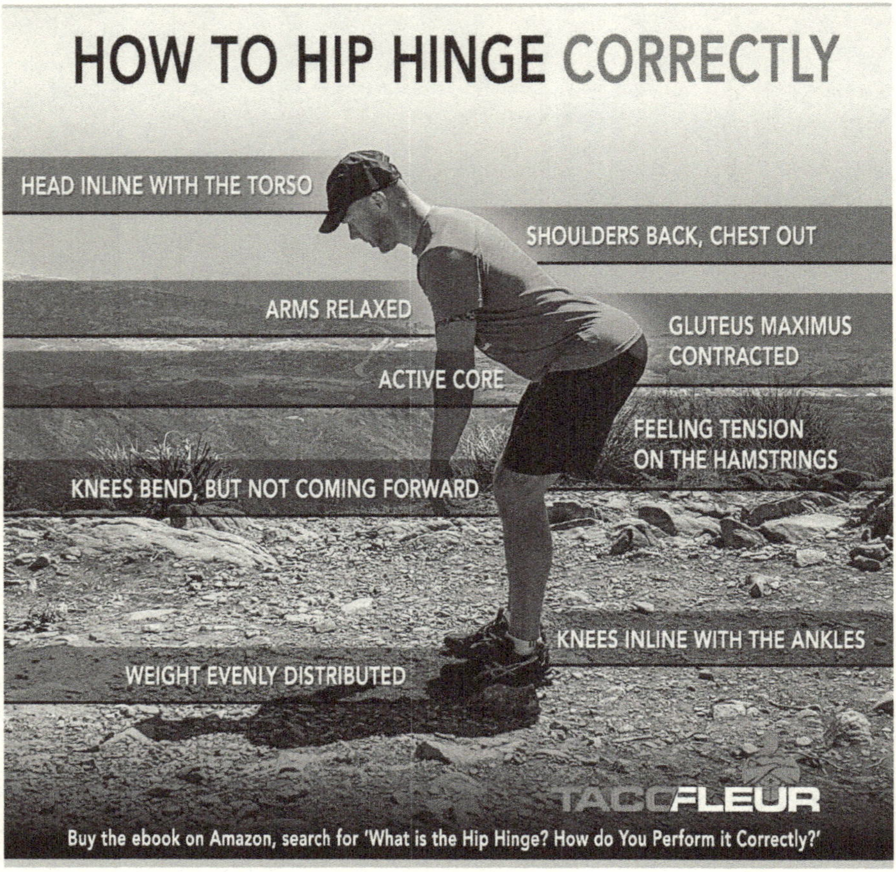

![How to Hip Hinge Correctly illustration]

[/Creative Commons License]

The above section between Creative Commons License is available as such, see below for the license.

Creative Commons License

Definition of the squat and hip hinge by Taco Fleur is licensed under a Creative Commons Attribution-NonCommercial-NoDerivatives 4.0 International License.

Based on a work at http://www.cavemantraining.com/caveman-bodyweight/true-definition-of-the-squat-and-hip-hinge-exercise/.

This means you can use that part freely with proper attribution and linking.

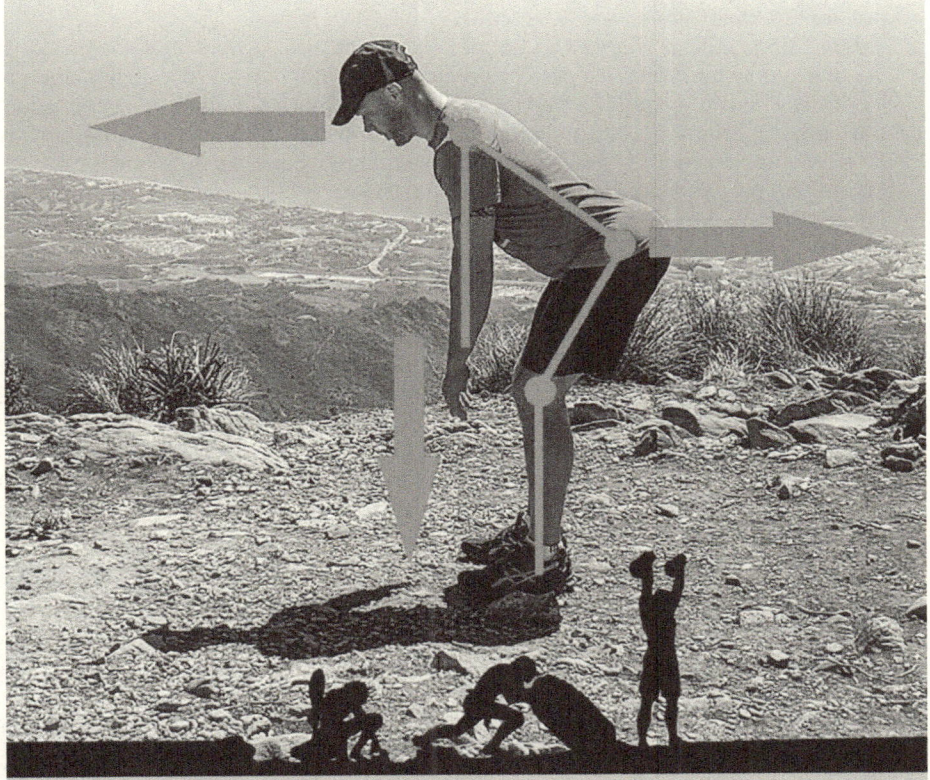

SWING SQUAT VS HIP HINGE STYLE

If you only just entered the kettlebell training world, you might not have heard about the squat vs hip hinge controversy. Like with anything, I suggest keeping an open mind.

"Performing a kettlebell swing squat style does not make you a bad trainer; performing an incorrect kettlebell swing squat style makes you a bad trainer. Performing a kettlebell swing 'any' style powered by the shoulders makes you a bad trainer."

-Taco Fleur

The hip hinge is the movement pattern with which the Russian swing was made popular, and anything that did not feature this movement was considered bad, but no more. The squat version is only bad when it's performed incorrectly and becomes damaging to the person performing the movement. If executed correctly, guess what? You're simply working and powering the movement with a different muscle group.

It's bad when you're doing a high number of kettlebell swings, using your shoulders and erector spinae to power the move, because your shoulders and erector spinae are more than likely not conditioned to perform this move one hundred times without getting injured. There is also nothing wrong with a shoulder raise if performed correctly with the appropriate weight and right amount of repetitions, and named correctly (i.e. not a "swing"). Watch a video here: www.youtube.com/watch?v=NI-uLguUQbeM

A kettlebell swing that looks like a squat is not bad – I repeat, it is not bad – it's simply a kettlebell swing squat style, assuming that the squat style is executed correctly and the arms are used as a pendulum. It's wrong when the person should be performing the hip hinge style, but is performing the squat style because their glutes are too weak to power the movement in the hip hinge.

A great way to spot if the shoulders are being used during the swing is when you see the kettlebell drooping at the top of the swing; if the kettlebell looks like an extension of the arm, it's more than likely that the swing was properly powered by the lower body.

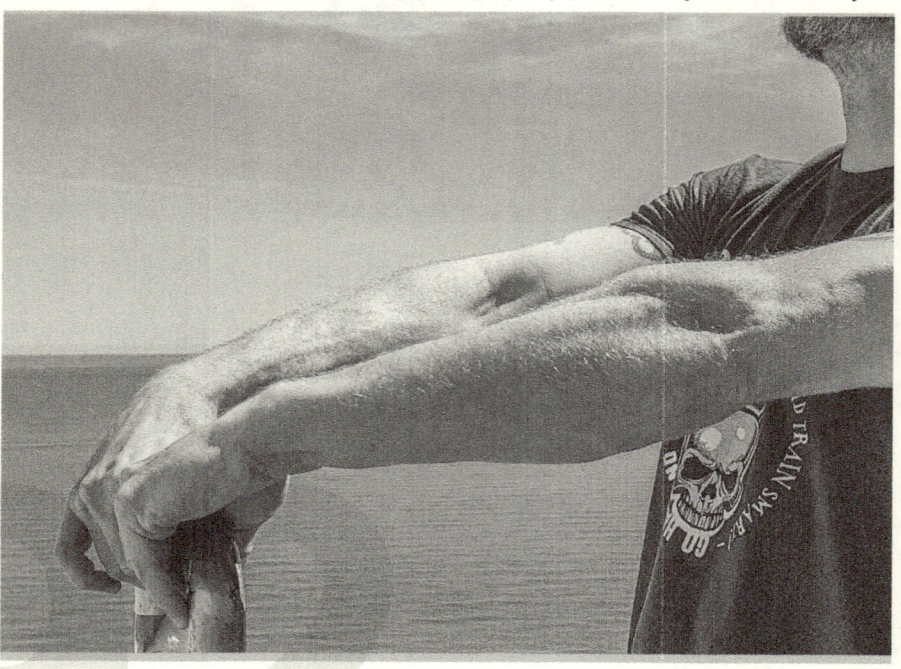

Drooping kettlebell

An exercise named "kettlebell swing" that has someone doing shoulder raises, is not necessarily bad if he/she intended to work the shoulders. It is, however, incorrectly named, and should be called "shoulder raise," "squat and shoulder raise," or "hip hinge and shoulder raise," depending on what he/she is doing.

Main Differences

- During the down phase of the hip hinge style, the weight is guided more toward the back; whereas with the squat style the weight is guided more towards the ground
- During the up phase of the hip hinge style, the weight is propelled more towards the front; whereas with the squat style the weight is propelled more towards the ceiling
- With the hip hinge style, the gluteus maximus mainly powers the swing; whereas with the squat style, the quadriceps also start powering the swing
- With the hip hinge style, the torso comes more toward the ground; whereas with the squat style, the torso stays more upright
- With the hip hinge style, the hamstrings get a good dynamic stretch on each rep; whereas with the squat style, the hip flexors get more of a stretch
- With the hip hinge style, the knees constantly remain above the ankles; whereas with the squat style the knees move forward and back

Correct Naming

✓ Kettlebell swing performed with a squat is called a "kettlebell swing squat style"

✓ Kettlebell swing performed with a hip hinge is called a "kettlebell swing hip hinge style"

✓ Kettlebell 'swing' performed with a shoulder raise is not called a swing but a "kettlebell shoulder raise"

What Not to Do

✗ Don't turn it into a deep squat (unless going into overhead)
✗ Don't turn it into a slow movement without explosiveness
✗ Don't lose form; keep the same tight and active posture as with the hip hinge
✗ Don't turn it into a bad squat, same principles as normal squatting apply

The reason I spend a considerable amount of time covering the squat vs hip hinge is because I'd like you to start thinking outside of the box: Think movement, safety and goals. If those are met, any intentional movement named correctly is okay. Last but not least, I highly recommend that anyone entering the kettlebell world first learn the hip hinge movement and fully understand how the arms should function during the swing, then progress to the squat-style swing. You'll also find that if you want to dip into the world of kettlebell sport, the squat style becomes more popular, even if not performed exactly the same way.

Now that we have covered the kettlebell swing, we're going to discuss another transitional movement. The double arm clean is a transitional movement which allows you to seamlessly move from a double arm swing into several different exercises.

The double arm clean is a transition from double hand grip to either horn grip or open hand horn grip. Your elbows should be tucked in, and the bell or handle should rest against your chest.

To complete the full movement, perform a double arm swing hip hinge style like you normally would, with the difference being that this time you want to keep the kettlebell close to your body as it comes up, rather than out and away. You do this by guiding it up plus in with the swing and by keeping the elbows tucked in.

You can move your hands from double hand grip to horn grip once the kettlebell is in front of your body by loosening the grip and sliding the hands up to the horns. You can choose to keep the thumbs over the index fingers while doing so to give you more confidence with this move. Once you become more secure with the movement, you can transition from double hand grip to open hand horn grip by letting go of the bell for a split second, moving the hands forward around the bell, and thumbs within the horns.

The open hand horn grip is the preferred grip, as the weight is more evenly distributed in the racking position. To return from a racking position into a swing, it's important to keep the weight close to the body going down and back; do not cast the weight out.

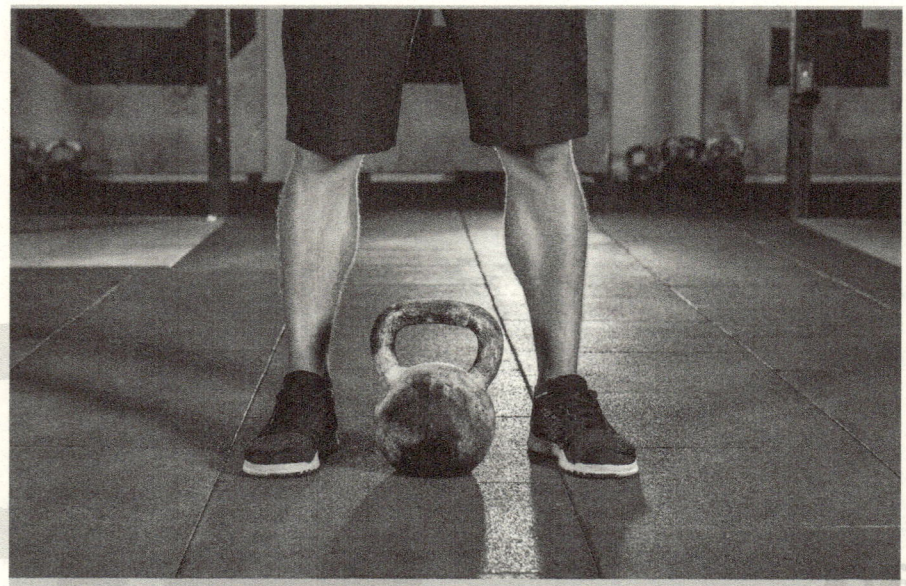

AMERICAN VS RUSSIAN SWING

The biggest difference between the American and Russian swing (AKA conventional kettlebell swing) is the height at which the kettlebell ends, the explosiveness required, and the involvement of the shoulders. There is also the fact that you simply shouldn't do an American swing with a very heavy weight.

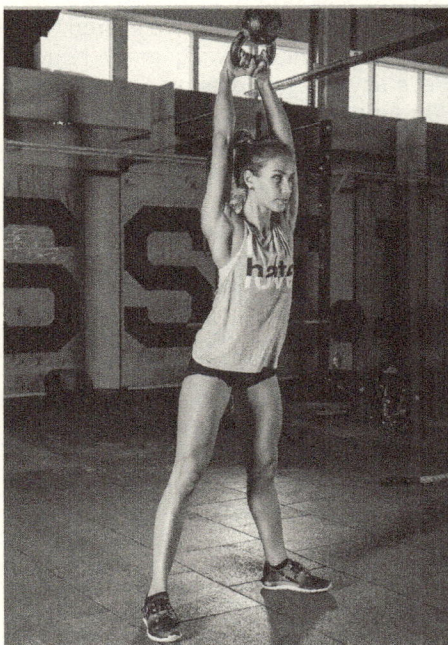
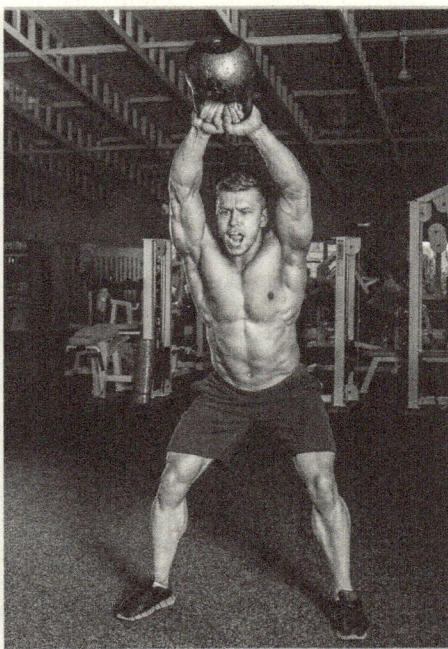

The American swing

THE PROBLEM WITH THE AMERICAN SWING

The American swing gets a bad rap within the kettlebell community because of the fact that CrossFit athletes are not taught the conventional swing first. Without this foundation, it encourages the athlete to primarily use their shoulders to do a lot of pulling, rather than hip and leg drive to get the weight up with the swing, hence the reason it's called American swing. When you consider that everything else in CrossFit when it comes to barbell work is pretty much pulling, it's quite easy for athletes to mistakenly apply that concept to the swing. This becomes a recipe for disaster and injury, especially with high reps and an awkward overhead position.

The second problem is that one needs good shoulder and thoracic mobility before being able to put the kettlebell overhead with such a narrow grip, and most people don't have this. Why force the shoulders into such an awkward position and a movement they are not ready for? You don't grab the barbell and do overhead squats with a narrow grip straight away, do you? No, you need to work up to that, and once you're able to do it, it becomes a show of mobility.

Context Is the Key

When it comes to programming, if you want to work the shoulders, throw some American swings in. Some people will say there are better ways to work the shoulders and this is true, but it's not always about what's better – we'd have some really boring programmes and clients would get bored quite quickly if it were.

I personally don't program American swings, but I can see how it would fit in a double arm kettlebell complex, like 3 x goblet squat, 3 x conventional swing, 3 x high swing, and 3 x American swing. By the way, I don't classify the high swing as an American swing; the high swing comes up just a bit higher than the conventional swing, in between shoulder height and above the head. I can also see the American swing as a progression to the KB snatch or regression for those who are injured.

If you want to swing really heavy, let's say 32kg or over, you should not do American swings. Of course Greg Glassman would say, "Most of our guys can easily do an American swing with 32kg," and in fact, I'd be really surprised if by "most of our guys" he was referring to most of the guys from all boxes across the world, because that sounds really unlikely and very dangerous for most of 'his guys.' The American swing movement standard requires the kettlebell to balance upside down above the head, with arms locked out. Do this with a heavy kettlebell, and you are gambling with injury upon each rep.

To be honest, I'm sick of the war between the American and Russian swing. Let's stop trying to make one look better than the other; they're both good after proper education and within the right context. The context you should consider when deciding to include one or both are:

- Safety
- Weight
- Repetitions
- Objectives
- Audience
- Experience

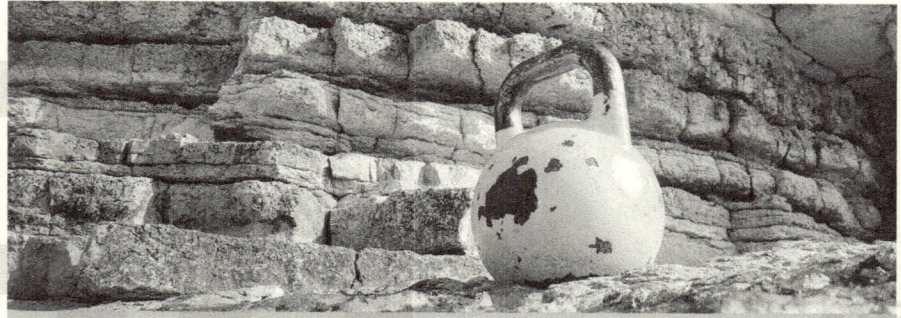

The following is what Greg Glassman, the founder of CrossFit, said about the American swing:

> "On first being introduced to the kettlebell swing, our immediate response was, 'why not go overhead?' Generally, we endeavour, somewhat reflexively, to lengthen the line of travel of any movement. why?
>
> There are two reasons. the first is somewhat intuitive. we don't do half rep pull-ups; we don't do half rep squats; and we don't do half rep push-ups. If there is a natural range of motion to any movement, we like to complete it. To do otherwise seems unnatural. We would argue that partial reps are neurologically incomplete. The second reason deals with some fundamentals of physics and exercise physiology.
>
> From physics we know that the higher we lift something, and the more it weighs, the more 'work' we are performing. Work is in fact equal to the weight lifted multiplied by the height we lift the object. Work performed divided by the time to completion is equal to the average 'power' expressed in the effort.
>
> Power is exactly identical to the exercise physiologist's 'intensity'. Intensity, more than any other measurable factor, correlates to physiological response. So more work in less time, or more weight moved farther in less time, is largely a measure of an exercise's potency.
>
> When we swing the kettlebell to overhead, the American swing, we nearly double the range of motion compared to the Russian swing, and thereby double the work done each stroke. For any given time period, the power would be equivalent only if the Russian swing rate was twice the American swing rate."

– Greg Glassman, founder of CrossFit

CrossFit made a huge mistake by focusing on the American swing for years, which has now caused a lot of injury* and inefficiency†, not only in the swing, but also their kettlebell snatch, simply because the foundation for the snatch and American swing had not been laid properly.

I also think it's a lot of bull to justify the American swing by saying it is more natural to complete. If that is the case, why do deadlifts at all? Why not complete it with a clean or snatch? Hold on... just because I don't agree with the above statement, does not mean I don't like the American swing; I'm just saying the above is not sufficient to justify it.

> "CrossFit is a great system, but they don't utilise kettlebells well because of a lack of qualified kettlebell instruction."
>
> *~ T.C., RKC*

I did not make the above comment, but I do agree with it. CrossFit is a great system, but it's not utilising kettlebells well due to the lack of qualified kettlebell instruction. This applies not just to CrossFit, but also to most gyms across the world. I also don't think the comment only referred to the American swing but to general kettlebell exercises employed within CrossFit boxes.

If you're doing Olympic lifting, you get

Olympic lifting coaches for teaching; if you're doing kettlebell training, you get…

The American swing is such a controversial topic in kettlebell training that I wanted to devote some time to it, and I've hopefully given you enough information to make a sound decision, and the ability to reply appropriately if ever caught in the American vs Russian swing war.

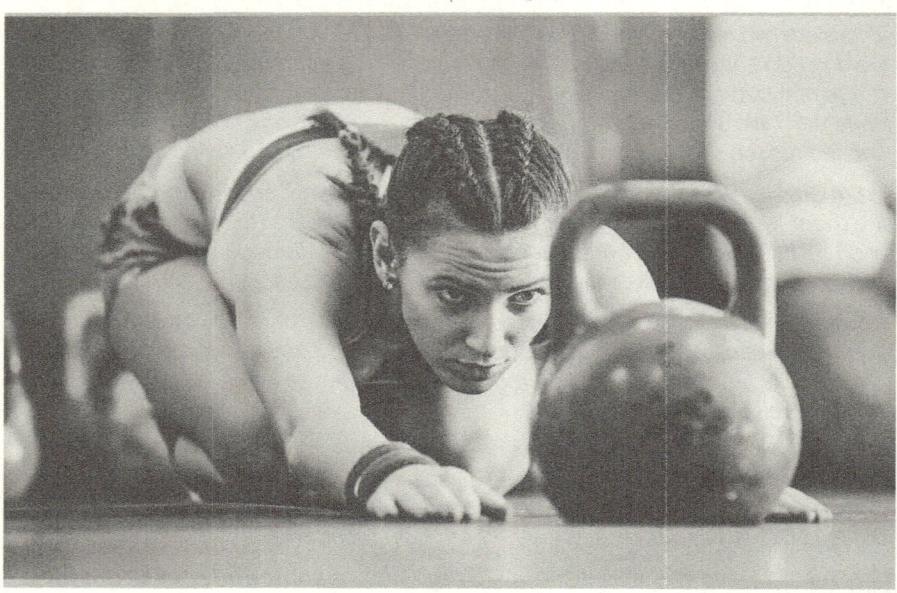

* when mentioning injury, I can only refer to which I've been witness to. There is no research paper that mentions the number of injuries. Therefore, make your own judgment on whether you see a lot of injuries due to this exercise.

* when mentioning inefficiency, again, it's based on what I've been witness to. There is no research paper that mentions the extent of inefficiency, nor whether there is any. Therefore, make your own judgment on whether you believe the foundation to make the exercises mentioned more efficient has been laid or not.

KETTLEBELL RACKING AND CLEANING

Racking a barbell or kettlebell is the process of putting a piece of equipment into a position where it can rest, preferably with little stress or resistance to the body. You can rack a barbell, sandbag, kettlebell, dumbbell, etc. To rack a kettlebell, you need to first clean it.

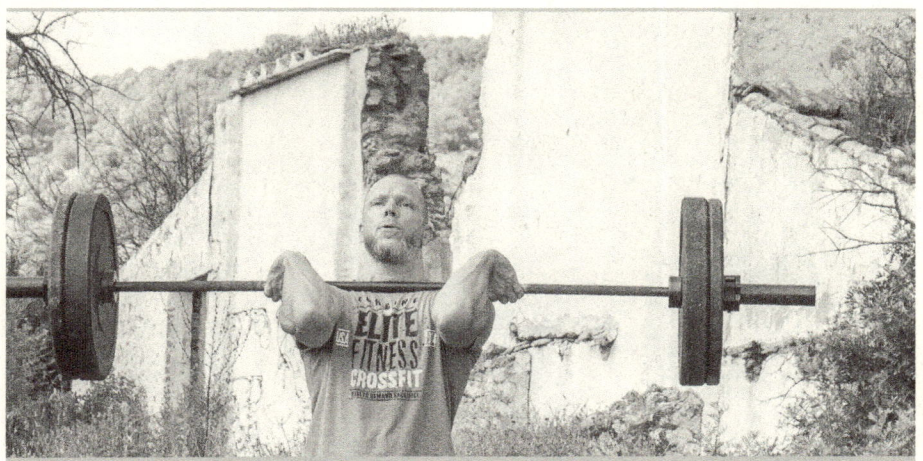

Barbell rack

"Finding your kettlebell racking position is not always easy. I have heard many different reasons that could be the problem, like, having breasts, not having the right body type, inflexibility, being overweight, etc. and yes, those could be valid excuses in some cases, but from my experience it's usually the trainer/teacher that does not know how to provide the proper progressions and cues for the student to find his/her racking position, or to make him/her fully aware of the position and its objectives."

-Taco Fleur

WHY RACK PROPERLY?

The main points why you should rack your kettlebell properly are:
- ✔ Conserve energy
- ✔ Be able to rest when required
- ✔ Allow for proper power transfer

Conserve energy by being able to relax the muscles more when in proper racking position, last longer in sets.

Being able to **rest** when required (i.e., when doing high-volume reps and not wanting to put the kettlebells down, as this would require more energy and time).

When doing jerks or push presses, **properly transfer the power** from the legs directly into the forearm through the elbow, rather than directing and losing power through the torso, shoulders, and elbow.

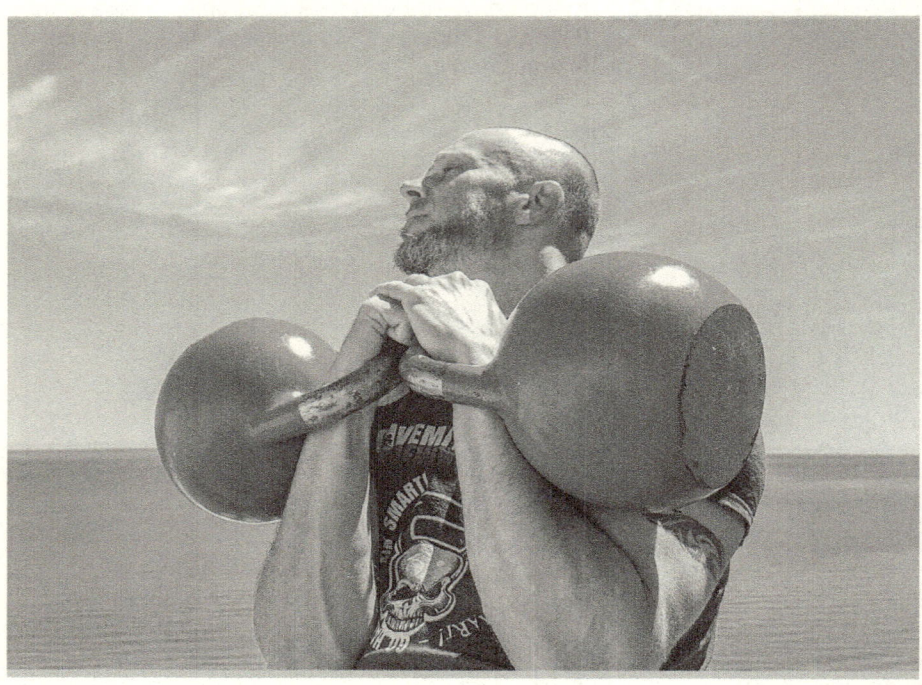

COMMON GRIPS IN RACKING

Following are the common grips used in the racking position:
- Racking grip
- Racking safety grip
- Flat hand grip
- Interlocking grip
- Stacking grip

Before delving deeper into racking, I will cover cleaning of a kettlebell.

KETTLEBELL CLEAN

Learning how to clean a kettlebell properly is an extremely important part of racking. All overhead presses require you to bring the weight from a lower position into racking position. Not knowing how to clean is a sure way to work out inefficiently and get injured. The clean is a beast that is tamed in detail in another book; before you can clean, you should know how to swing; before you can swing you should know how to hip hinge.

Make sure you check out our book on Amazon, The Kettlebell Swing: Amazingly Simple, but Extremely Detailed, and the precursor Hip Hinge Movement—How do you perform it correctly?.

I highly recommend you read these two books, as it's simply too much to cover here, but I do want to introduce the most basic clean you should learn for safely picking up kettlebells, the assisted clean.

ASSISTED CLEAN

Learning the assisted clean properly is vitally important, because literally everything you do as a beginner will build upon this. If you get it wrong, it's going to take a long time to unlearn bad habits and get it right. Everyone working with kettlebells will need to clean a kettlebell and rack it.

The following are dot points to cover the assisted clean. Please watch the video for additional details:

1. Stand in position for a squat
2. Squat
3. Brace your core
4. Arm straight
5. Employ hook grip
6. Lift
7. Full hip and knee extension
8. Assist with the other hand
9. Corkscrew
10. Hand insert
11. Handle 45°
12. Rack
13. Assist
14. Reverse corkscrew
15. Hook grip
16. Hang
17. Squat

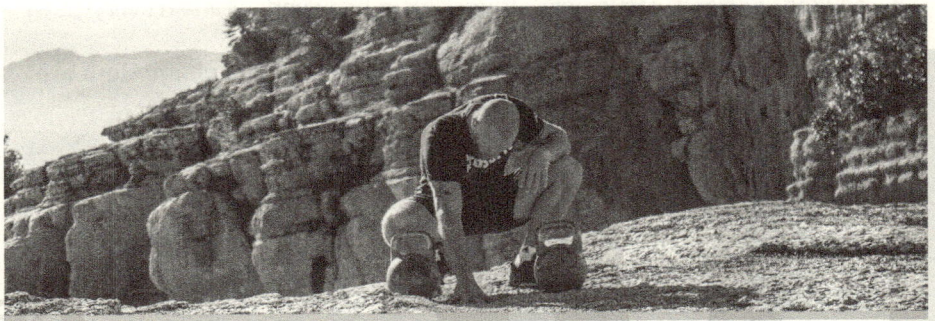

Video: Kettlebell Training For Complete Beginners

 youtube.com/watch?v=BniipxsR-Bl

Video: Kettlebell Fundamentals Assisted Clean

 bit.ly/youtube-assisted-clean

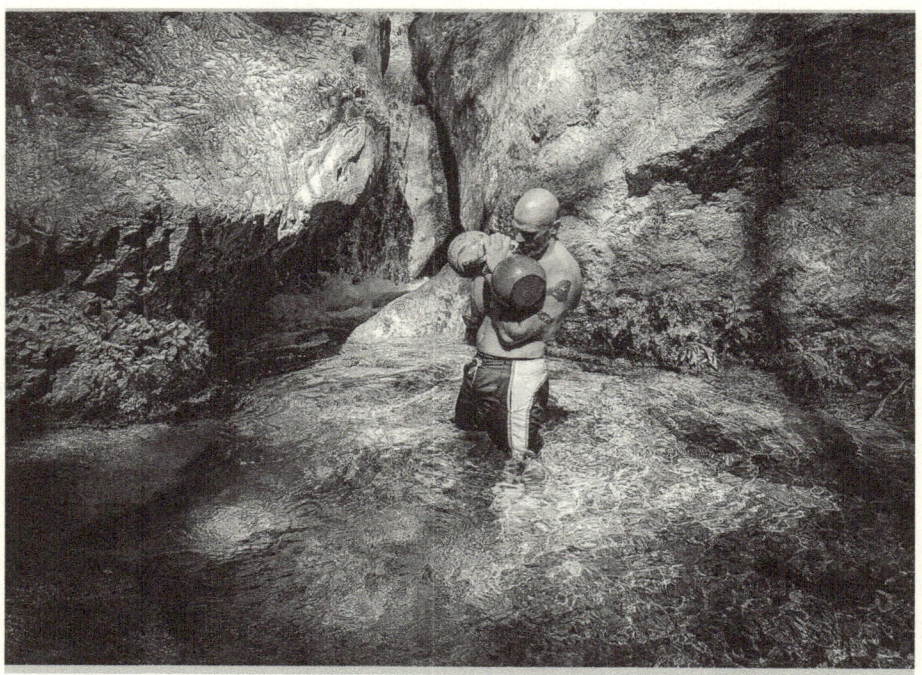

Why Is It Called a Clean?

Here's an interesting one for you, as I know you've been wondering about the name – yes you have, admit it! The movement is called a "clean", because it requires a clean movement, free from irregularities, smoothly and skilfully performed. If you lift your barbell or kettlebell up and the movement is interrupted, or the equipment bangs on your body parts, it wasn't very clean.

In kettlebell training, there are different variations of the clean. Here are some of the most common ones:
- Assisted clean (AKA cheat clean)
- Dead clean
- Dead swing clean
- Swing clean
- Hang clean

Exercise Equipment

There are different types of exercise equipment with which one can perform a weight-lifting clean, some of them being:
- Kettlebells
- Olympic Bars
- Sand Bags
- Aqua Bags
- Wall Balls
- Dead Balls
- Dumbbells

Type of Cleans
- Dead clean, the weight starts dead on the ground without momentum before being cleaned
- Hang clean, the weight is hanging from the ground before being cleaned
- Swing clean, the weight is swinging before being cleaned
- Dead swing clean, the weight is dead on the ground and pulled into a swing before being cleaned
- Assisted clean, the weight is cleaned with assistance from another person or the other hand

AMBIGUITY OF CLEANS

Not calling a specific clean what it is creates a lot of ambiguity and confusion in the fitness industry, which can be avoided by getting specific with the naming and using the correct name when explaining and programming cleans for your clients.

COMMON CLEAN MISTAKE

The most common mistake made while cleaning a weight is that the athlete uses the upper body to get the weight to a racking position (i.e., curling it up with upper-body strength only, mainly the biceps). This is especially noticeable with beginners using a weight that is too light, in which case they are unaware of the concept of using the stronger muscles of the body (legs) to power the clean. They will (understandably) think, "This is so light that there is no need to make it complicated."

This is where a good trainer comes in and explains that the lighter weight is used to master the exercise execution, and trying to curl a heavy weight with the upper body can become impossible or even cause injury.

WEAKEST POINT

Most types of cleans, no matter what exercise equipment with which they are performed, usually challenge the trapezius, posterior chain muscles, and grip. With high reps the grip is usually the weakest point, thus your clean is only as good as your grip strength.

CLEAN VARIATIONS

Receiving the Kettlebell

You can change the way you receive the kettlebell. Usually this is with everything locked out, but you can also initiate the clean and receive it in squat position, a pull powered by the legs and then coming under the kettlebell with a squat; great for extremely heavy kettlebells. You can also receive it in a split lunge, etc.

Next you can start adding alternating reps, and finally you can work with one or two kettlebells. With all that said, lets list the variations:

- Single arm assisted clean
- Single arm squat dead clean
- Alternating arm squat dead clean
- Double kettlebell squat dead clean
- Single arm hip hinge dead clean
- Alternating arm hip hinge dead clean
- Double kettlebell hip hinge dead clean
- Single arm dead swing clean
- Alternating arm dead swing clean
- Double kettlebell dead swing clean
- Double arm one kettlebell dead swing clean
- Single arm hang clean
- Alternating arm hang clean
- Double kettlebell hang clean
- Single arm swing clean
- Alternating arm swing clean
- Double arm one kettlebell swing clean
- Double kettlebell swing clean
- Single arm dead diagonal squat clean
- Single arm dead diagonal hip hinge clean

- Single arm dead staggered squat clean (knee is past the ankle, loading the quads more)
- Single arm dead lunge clean (knee does not travel past the ankle)
- Single arm lawnmower clean (quads are fully loaded)

If I indicated the way you receive the kettlebell as another variation, we could turn this list into 45 kettlebell clean variations, but let's not go there… instead, check out the book Master The Kettlebell Clean, it will cover everything you need to master the clean.

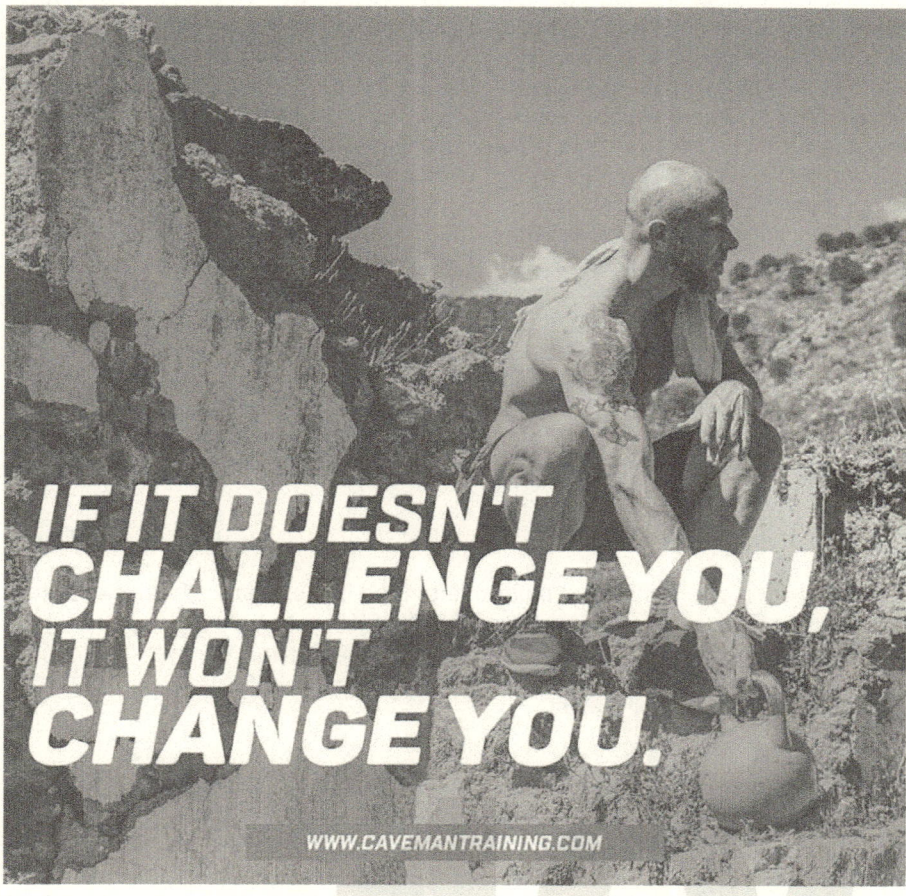

SWING CLEAN

Most people will refer to this simply as the "clean", due to this being the most popular variation of the clean, but I suggest to use its full name when possible.

When you perform the swing clean, you still need to execute the movement as if you were going to perform a kettlebell swing. You start with your back swing upon which your forearm and elbow make connection, and normally disconnect in the frontal plane (kettlebell is in front of you). When you do a swing clean, however, on the upward arc, you need to keep the elbow tight or close to your mid-section, hips, or ribs, all depending on what's comfortable for you and how your body is designed.

When the kettlebell is approximately above or in line with your elbow, you need to focus on opening up your hand and let the kettlebell come up through the power generated and perform a hand insert. You do this by lightly punching the open hand up into the kettlebell handle at the corner, which is located between the horn and handle of the kettlebell; at the same time, you need to focus on twisting the hand to make sure the kettlebell travels around the hand and does not flip over the hand. This is to stop the bell from producing friction in the palm of the hand and banging on the wrist.

On the down phase of the clean, you need to choose the shortest path down and back between the legs. Rotate your wrist to guide the handle from the 45 degree resting position on your palm to back into the hook grip, all of this preferably while reducing contact and friction between the handle and your hand. In other words, bump it from the resting position into hook grip.

Think about the whole process of cleaning the kettlebell up as guiding the kettlebell all the way; there is not one point where you're not guiding the kettlebell to where you want it to end up. You want a clean, smooth movement. If you let the kettlebell choose its own path, you will end up with injuries, pain, or simply a sloppy-looking clean.

Friction

Friction between the handle and palm of the hand is the main culprit for calluses or ripped skin. There are several causes for this friction:

- ✘ Tight grip during the clean
- ✘ Kettlebell flipping over the fist
- ✘ Casting the kettlebell out
- ✘ No transition into hook grip

Bruises

The main area where people get bruises is on the forearm or near the shoulder. This is due to the impact of an improperly guided kettlebell:

- ✘ Kettlebell flips over the fist
- ✘ Receiving the kettlebell out too far from the body

✗ Receiving the kettlebell too high
✗ Elbow is disconnected from the body

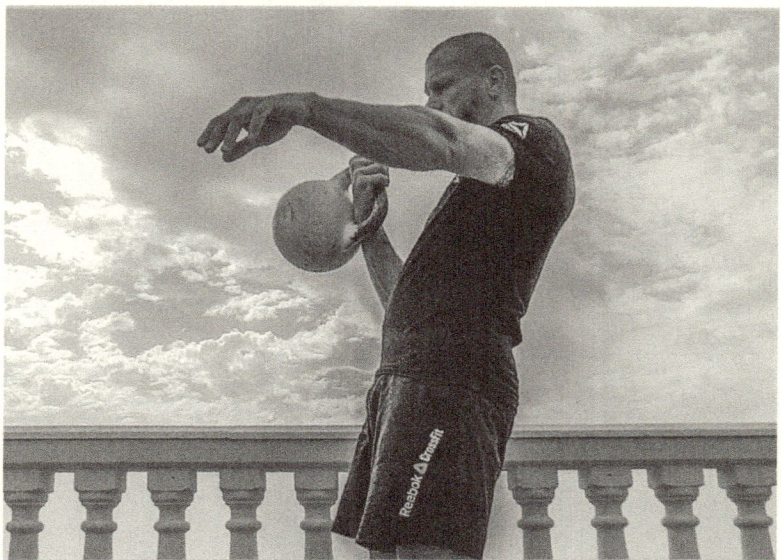

Start in racking position.

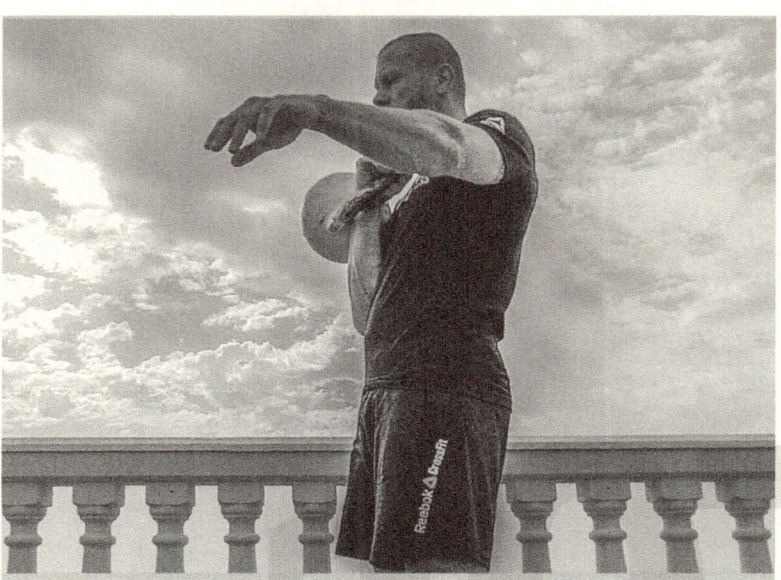

Push yourself away from the kettlebell.

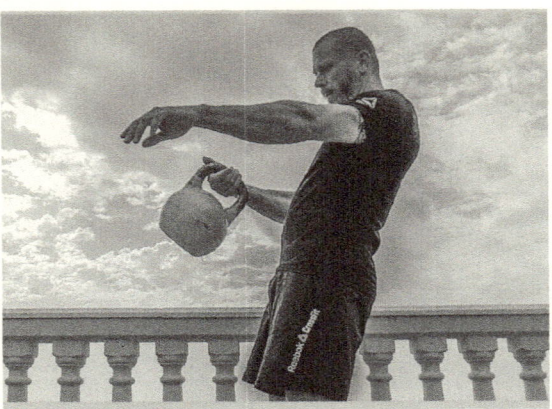

Catch the kettlebell in hook grip.

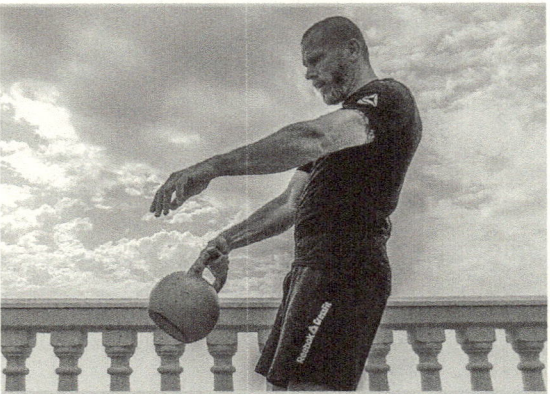

Delay hip hinging.

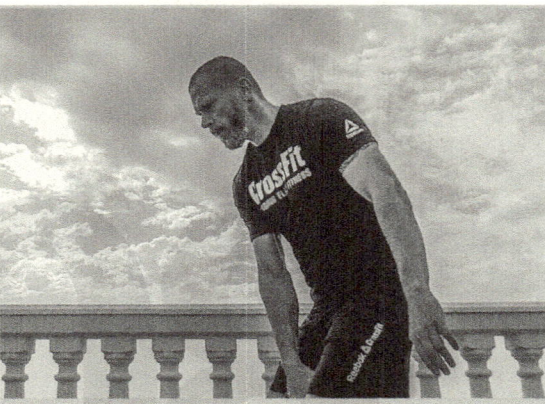

Hip hinge.

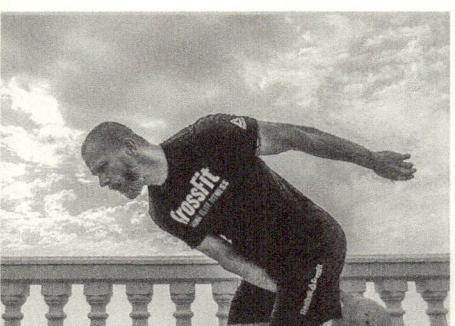 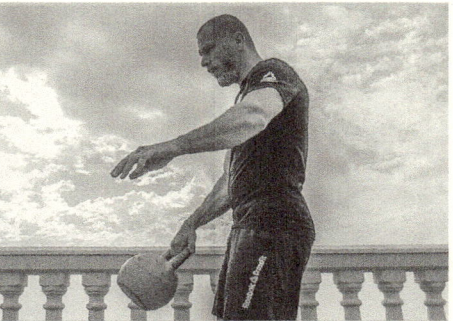

Come back up, with the elbow close to the body.

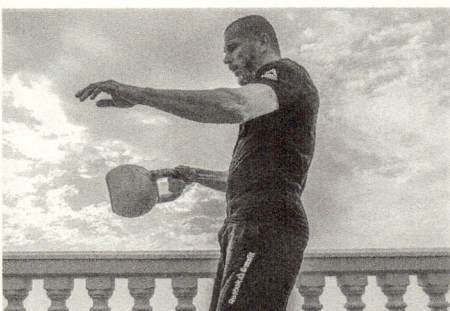 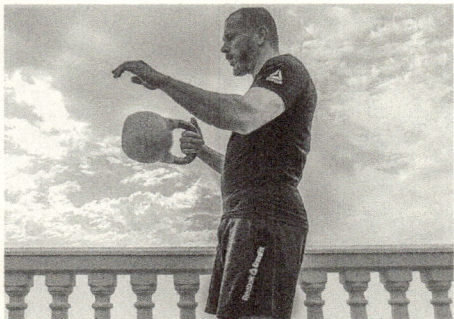

Open up and insert.

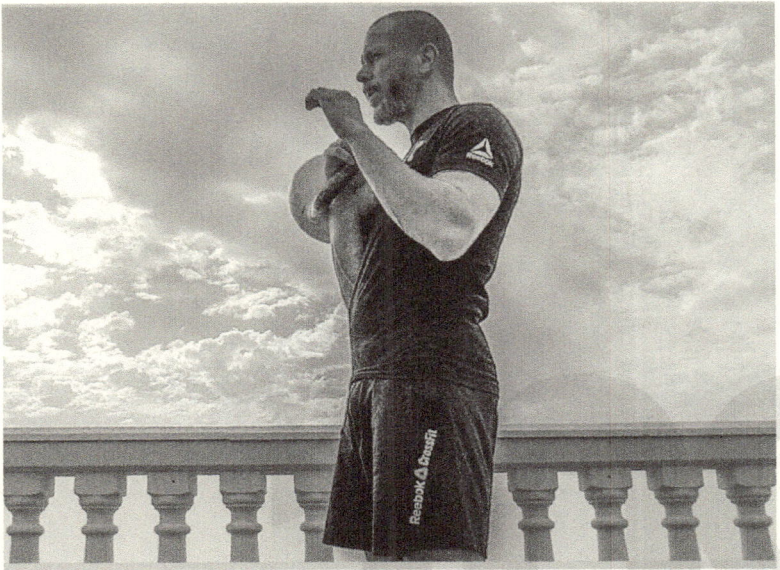

Video: youtube.com/watch?v=M9IGVGTWH_4

Kettlebell flipping over the fist and banging. Incorrect technique.

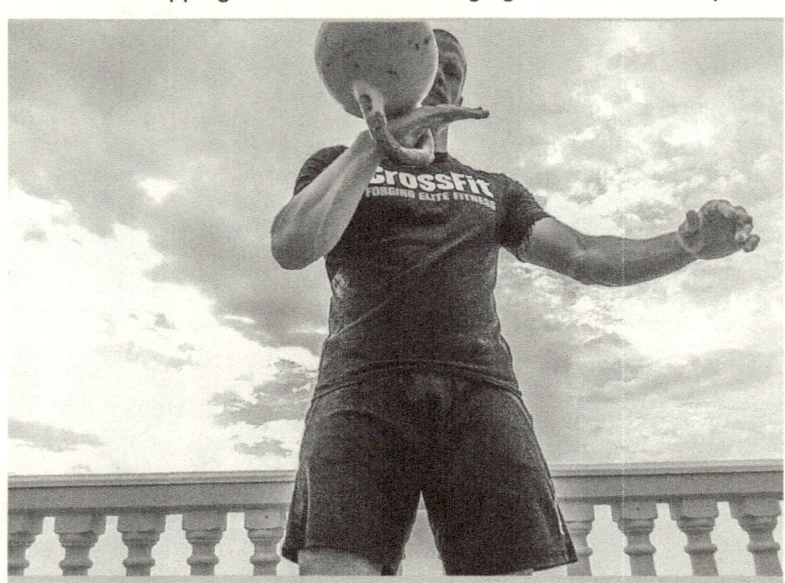

Produces bruising, and other pains.

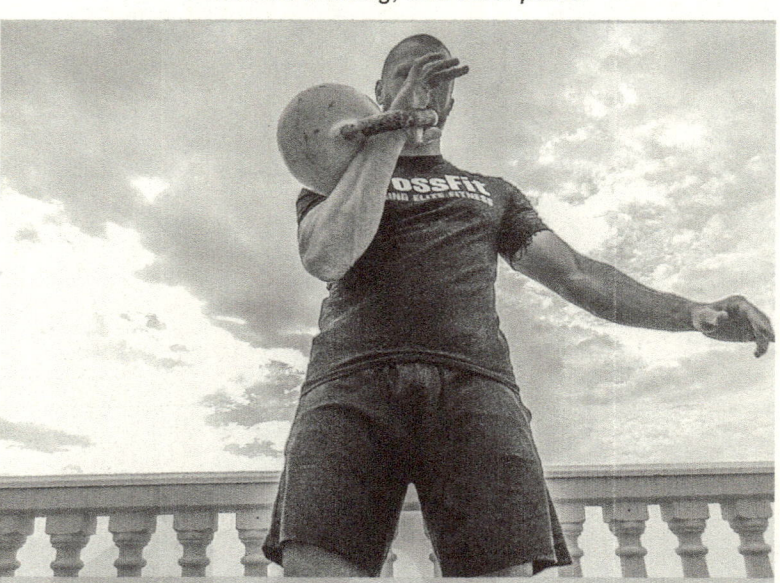

DEAD CLEAN

The dead clean is a great type of clean to learn, maybe even before the swing clean if your goal is pressing and other overhead and racked exercises. To perform the dead clean:

1) Come into a squat
2) Kettlebell positioned between the feet
3) Grab the handle in the corner
4) Brace the chest, shoulders, and traps
5) Pull the lats down to secure the shoulder into its socket
6) Activate the core
7) Create slight tension between the kettlebell and yourself
8) Start pulling up towards the ceiling
9) The kettlebell should travel in one straight path from the ground to racking position
10) Accelerate the pull all while avoiding the shoulder from being pulled down
11) Fully straighten the knees and hips before bending the elbow, or as close to it as possible
12) Open the hand and insert it into the handle
13) Find your racking position; type of rack depends on your transition
14) Start corkscrewing the palm reverse direction
15) Bring the elbow up to avoid jarring the shoulder
16) Bend the knees and bring the kettlebell to the ground in a controlled manner
17) Let the legs take the impact of lowering the weight
18) Kettlebell dead on the ground before attempting another repetition

Remember that it's going to be a bit different for everyone. In the end you need to understand the form and technique, and you will be able to make your own adjustments to shape the perfect clean for you.

ONE BELL RACKING POSITION

Following are some points and tips that I employ to help my students find their one bell racking position easily. The first step is to find the racking position without weight using the following moves and cues to practise.

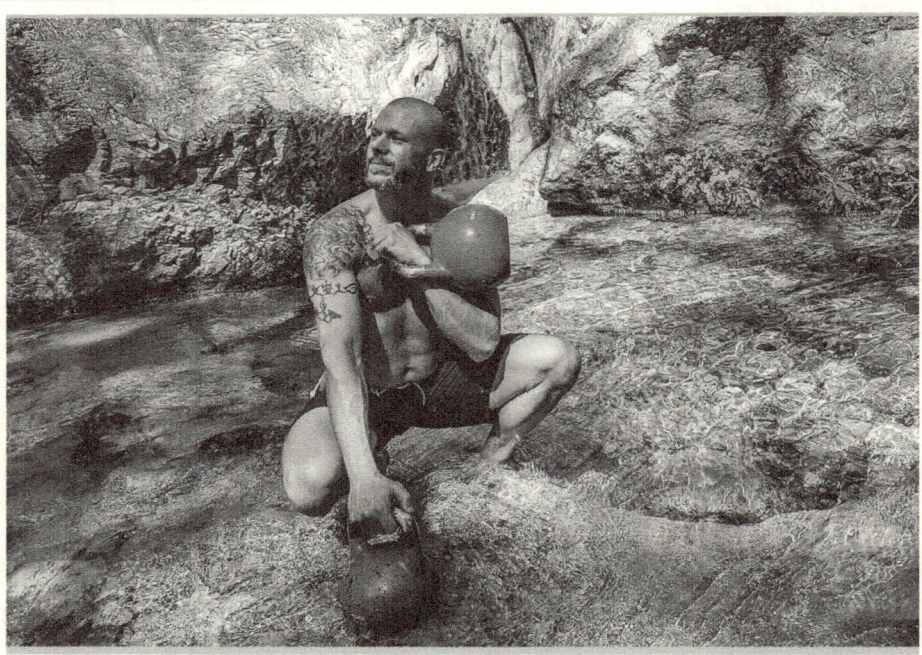

BODYWEIGHT RACKING PRACTISE

1) Stand straight in a neutral position
2) Bend one arm to bring the hand to the chest
3) Keep the elbow tucked in
4) Loosen the hips
5) Squeeze the glutes to create hip extension (not lumbar extension)
6) Fill the chest with a deep breath of air
7) Breath out, release all the air while crunching forward
8) Crunch to the side
9) Push the hip slightly towards the side on which you're racking
10) Make adjustments if the forearm is not directly vertically aligned with the leg

SPINE POSITION FOR RACKING

The upper part of the torso needs to come away from its natural position, which would be in line with the hips in neutral standing position. Why? Consider two heavy kettlebells in racking position with your body being in a normal neutral standing position. All the weight would be pulling forward; this would keep the body under tension, wear out the biceps, and provide you with no rest.

See infographic below.

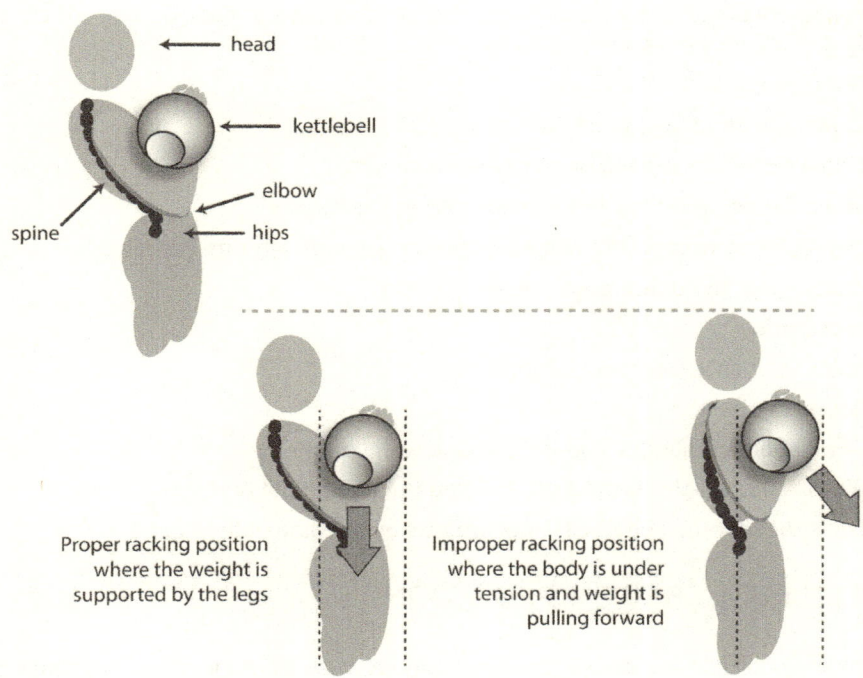

Now consider the spine making way for the kettlebells, allowing the weight to be placed above the hips and supported by the legs. *See infographic below.*

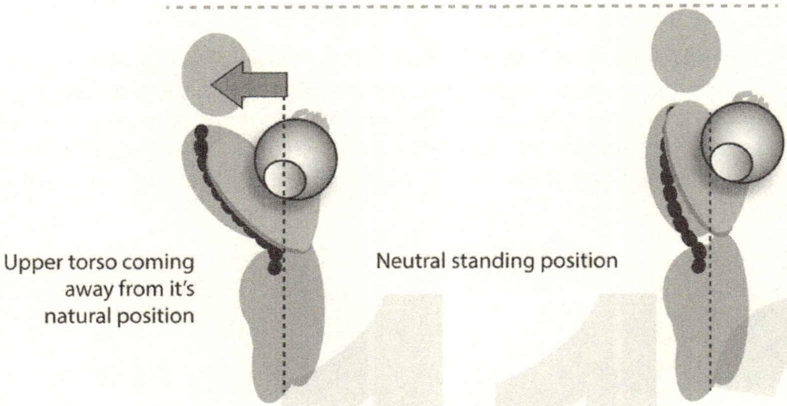

RACKING POINTS AND CUES

Following are some racking points and cues you can use to find yourself or help a student find a proper racking position:

- The hips are soft not locked
- Glutes are squeezed to create hip extension
- Elbow resting on the hip or as close as possible
- Straight wrist when the bell is resting on the forearm
- Slightly bend wrist when the bell is resting between forearm and biceps
- Handle at a 45 degree angle within the palm
- Loose grip
- Relax your shoulders and trapezius
- Round the back
- Think about creating a side-on S shape with your body
- With proper weight distribution, the forearm should not hurt
- The space for the kettlebell is not created by bending at the hips

KETTLEBELL RESTING POSITION

The kettlebell can rest on the forearm or between the forearm and biceps; this is determined by the angle between the hand and the chest. If the hand is more toward the chest, the bell will be resting more on the forearm. If the hand comes more away from the chest—increasing the angle—the bell will be resting more between the forearm and biceps. Women with larger breasts will need to rest the kettlebell between the forearm and biceps plus increase the angle.

Most trainers recommend to lock the knees out, which makes sense; let the weight rest on the skeletal system and not the muscles. I find this doesn't always work for me personally, and I can find more comfortable positions with my knees slightly bent. Knees slightly bent also helps if you're not very flexible at the hips, allowing you to move the weight above the feet without great hip flexibility. Use what works best for you.

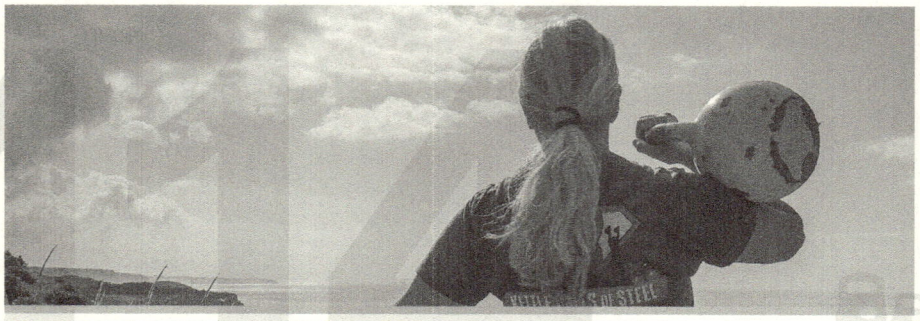

THE RACKING CONCEPT

In the end, it's about understanding the main concepts of racking. Do what you can to get the maximum benefit from these concepts, and you are doing well.

- Let the skeletal system take as much of the weight as possible
- Let your legs do the work

With all that said, it should be stated that there is not one position that works for all. Everybody is different; adjustments need to be made, and some people just won't be able to get a perfect racking position. Some might need to employ a racking position with a stacking grip (two kettlebells) and rest on one hip by leaning off to one side. In the end, as long as the effort is made and the points are understood, you will be fine.

If you can't obtain a good racking position no matter what, you should consider resting in overhead lock-out.

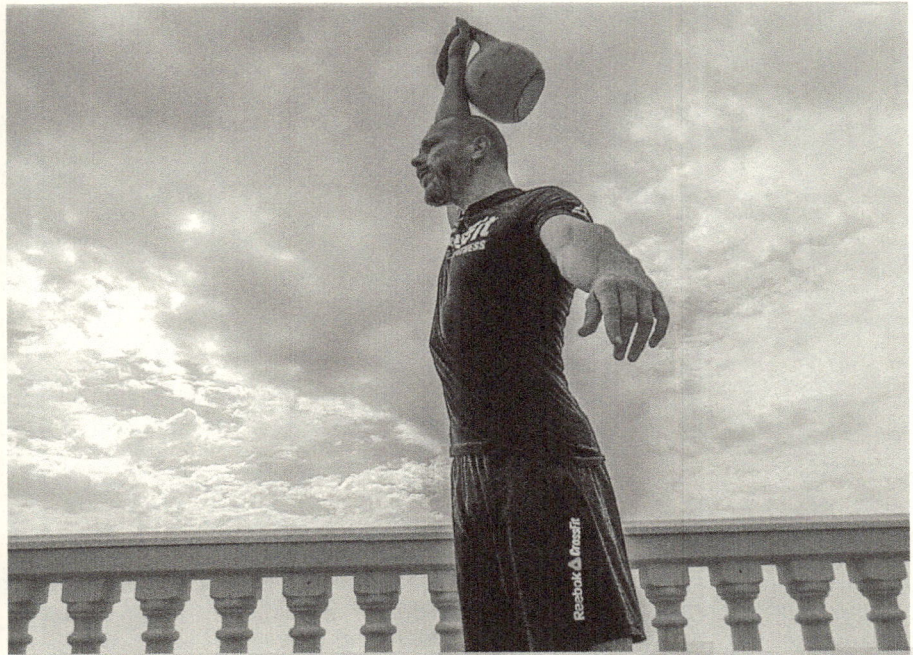

RACKING TYPES AND RACKING FOR FEMALES

Cradle Racking Position

The cradle rack is a position where the bell rests in the cradle of your biceps and forearm, and your hand is turned away from the chest. This is also the best racking position for females with ample breasts; the larger the breasts, the further away the palm should turn away from the chest. Furthermore, this position is also good if you have forearm bruises or other problems, as the weight is shared through support from the biceps; hence, only half the weight is on your forearm. Last but not least, the cradle racking position is also the most efficient for the front press, as the weight is directly above your forearm and not pulling to one side. The weight is closer to the end point, not only vertically, but also in front. We are talking inches, but inches start to count with heavy weight and high-volume reps.

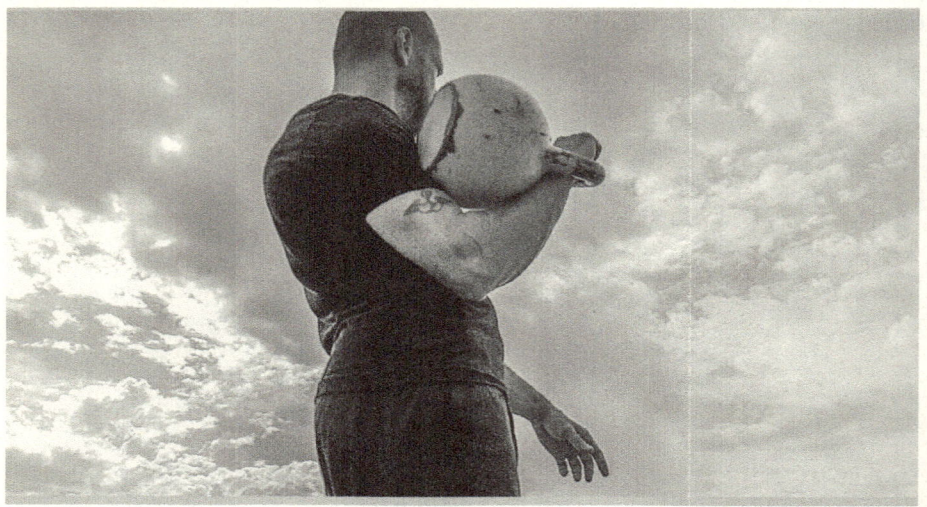

Cradle racking position

Hybrid Racking Position

I've had quite a few people ask me what the best kettlebell racking position for women in CrossFit is. Whether you do CrossFit, kettlebell training, or kettlebell sport, the concept is all the same. The cradle rack is the best position for women with large breasts. The hybrid rack is positioned between chest and cradle.

Chest Racking Position

The chest rack is the most common racking position in kettlebell training, where the hand is more placed to the centre line of the chest, and the bell rests more on the forearm.

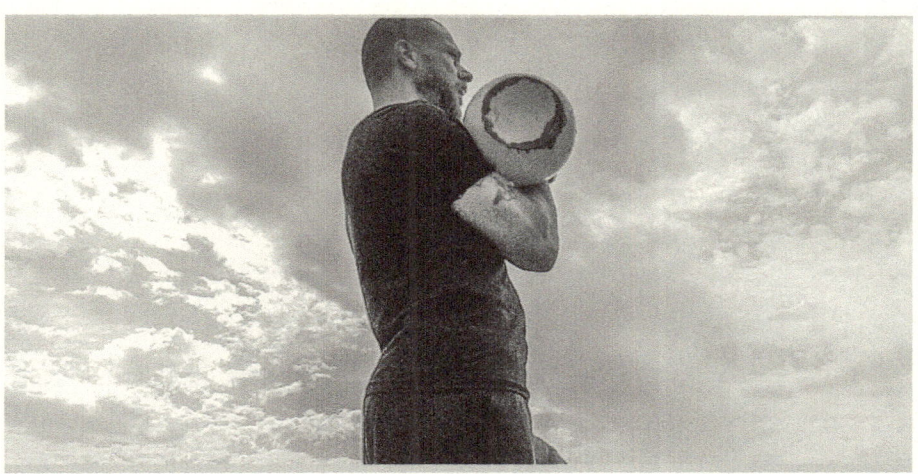

Chest racking position

Shoulder Racking Position

I named this position the shoulder rack; this racking position is certainly not something you see employed often in kettlebell training, and certainly not in KB sport, apart from a split second before entering the racking position at the front. But you can carry your kettlebells around in this position for walking drills, or even when having to move your kettlebell.

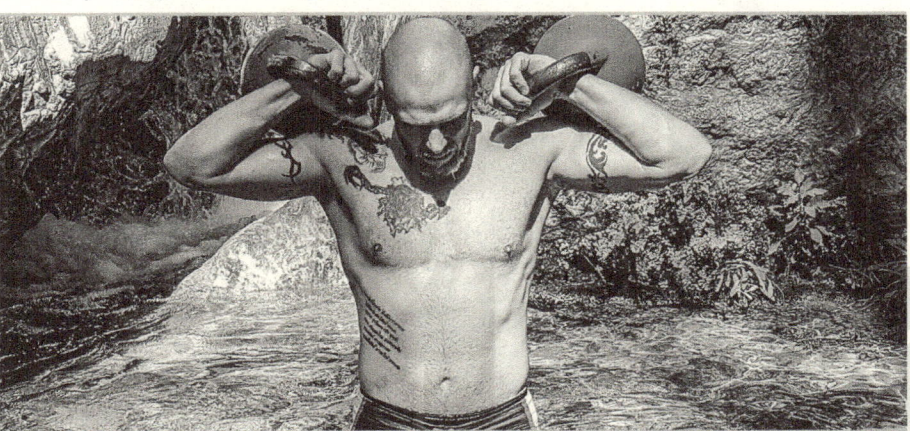

Shoulder racking position

Trap Racking Position

I named this position the trap rack, and again this is not a position that is seen in conventional methods of training, but this is Cavemantraining, so we have to be unconventional and do what others don't. It's a great position to perform back squats in. You can see a video of this in the article "14 Kettlebell Squat Variations": https://www.youtube.com/watch?v=jku4gGlwuSo

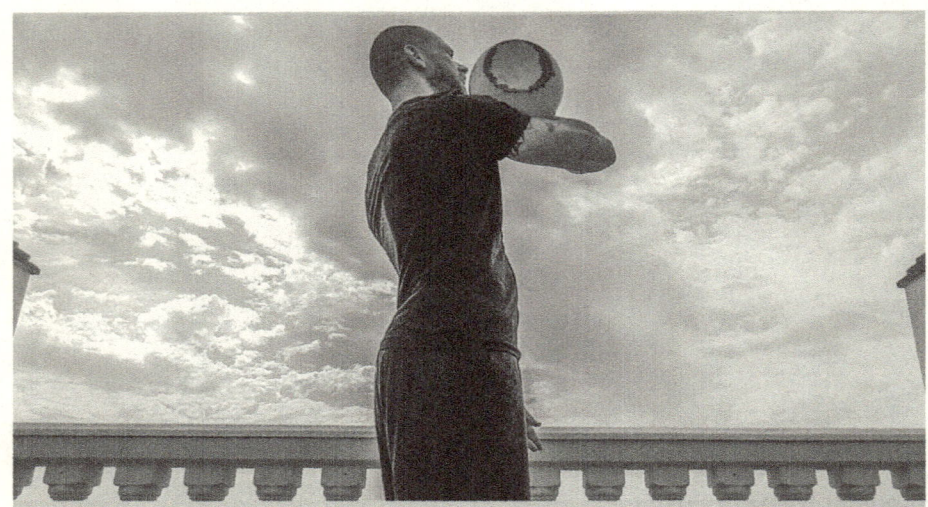

Incorrect rack

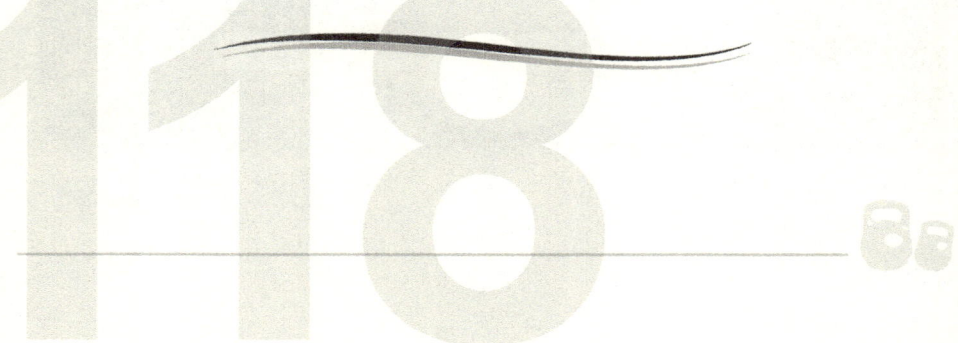

Step 1. racking position. Step 2. crunch. Step 3. hip extension (not lumbar extension).

KETTLEBELL PAIN

Following are some of the major causes that produce pain or discomfort when training with kettlebells:

✓ **Jarring**
Jarring (a quick, sharp, sudden movement) movement of the kettlebell causing shoulder pain

✓ **Friction**
Friction between the kettlebell handle and the hand, causing calluses or ripping skin

✓ **Impact**
Banging of the kettlebell on the forearm, causing bruising

✓ **Pressure**
Pressure of the weight in one place, rather than distributed

✓ **Incorrect technique**
Coming too low with the kettlebell, putting undue pressure on the lower back

✓ **Prolonged muscle tension causing strain can lead to tendinopathy**
Performing high-volume reps while unconditioned or with incorrect technique

MUSCLE ACHES

If you are properly recruiting the right muscles in a swing and you just started training with kettlebells, some muscle ache in the hamstrings, lower-back muscles, and gluteals is quite normal. The same goes for any other exercise that you do correctly but have just started or increased your weight or repetitions on, but you should be able to identify and differentiate between muscle ache and muscle pain. The first is quite normal, but the latter is the one you want to avoid at all costs.

The following are some of the common symptoms of pain and discomfort people can experience:

CALLUSES

Calluses are hardened layers of skin which may appear greyish or yellowish that develop when your skin tries to protect itself against friction and pressure. The pressure and friction cause the skin to die and form a hard, protective surface. Any type of pressure or friction applied to the callus can cause pain, and if continued can rip the skin.

No matter how much attention I pay to doing things right, I develop calluses. I have them from pull-ups, barbell dead lifts, etc. It's important to remove calluses; you can do this with a scraper, hot water, and pumice stone. Also use coconut or other oils during the night to soften the affected areas. Don't overdo it with chalking of the hands; instead use light chalk only when needed (i.e., when doing high reps, snatches, clean and jerks, etc.).

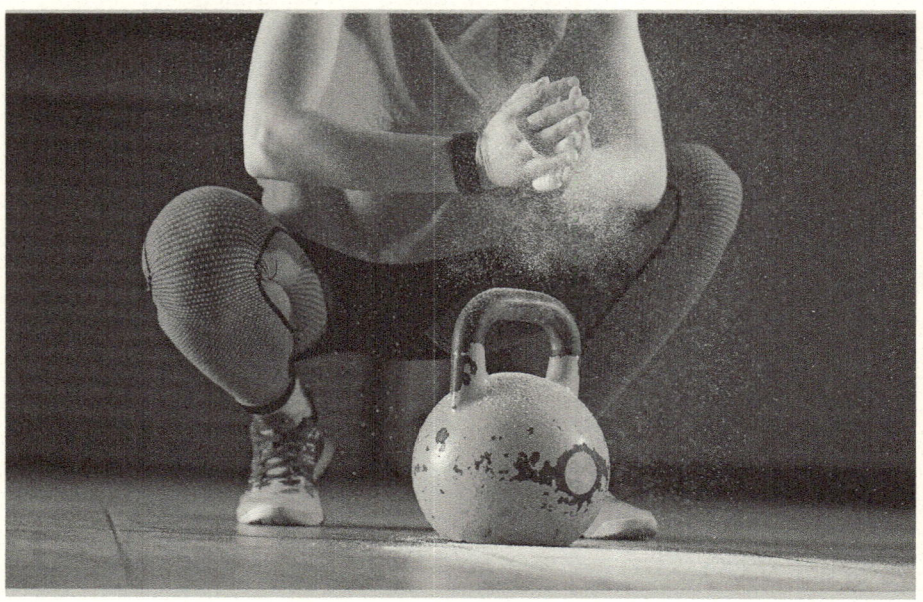

FOREARM PAIN AND BRUISES

Forearm pain and bruises are usually the cause of kettlebells hitting the forearm with more force than they should when landing on your forearm. If the kettlebell is banging on your forearm, it could be due to the kettlebell traveling over the fist rather than inserting the hand and rotating it (corkscrew). It could also be due to the kettlebell coming up too high and then landing on the forearm with a lot of force. I should mention that a little bruising is common for beginners, even when getting all the movements right; after all, the forearm is not used to the pressure from a heavy object and needs to be conditioned. Muscle pain and cramps in the forearms is usually a sign of holding the kettlebell too tightly.

Following are some common causes for forearm pain/pressure and bruises:
- ✗ Flexed wrist
- ✗ Weak wrist
- ✗ Fingers gripping tight around the handle
- ✗ Hand inserted in middle of handle
- ✗ Cleaning and banging
- ✗ Letting the bell rest on the forearm

If you really need to, get yourself some wrist guards or sweat bands, but personally I find it best to get conditioned and focus on correct technique.

If you get to a stage where the weights you're lifting are very heavy and you're doing high reps, go and get those wrist guards!

Here are some techniques that will reduce or prevent forearm issues:
- ✓ Keep the wrist straight
- ✓ Proper hand insertion
- ✓ Push the thumb up
- ✓ Maintain close to vertical forearm

An incorrect insert where the hand is in the middle of the horn will place the middle of bell on the forearm, which will create more pressure.

A proper hand insert is where the top corner of the handle is positioned on the webbing between your thumb and index finger; from there the handle is resting on the ball of the thumb, the thumb is pushing up through a slight but natural lateral wrist rotation, the bottom corner of the handle is past the heel of your palm, and the bottom horn is resting against the side of your forearm without causing pressure. The weight is distributed across the ball of your thumb and heel of your palm, and your forearm is nearly free from pressure.

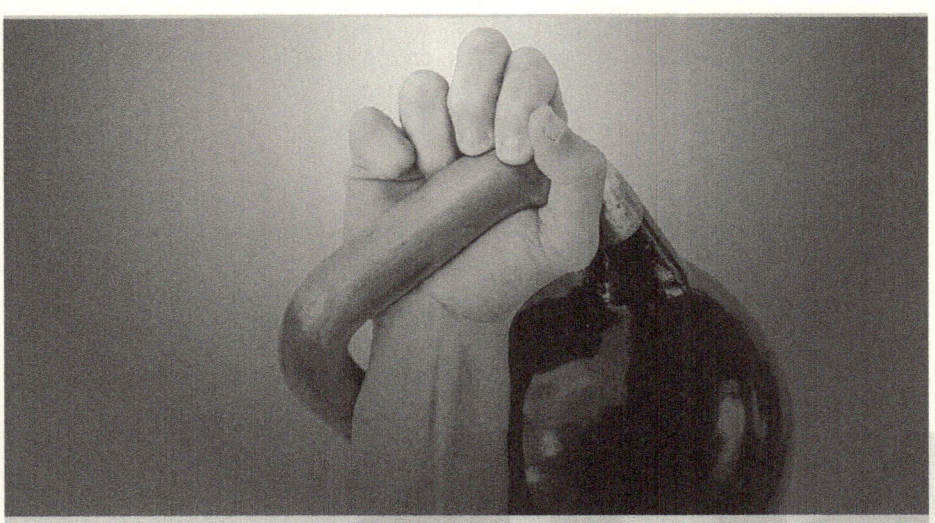

Due to the design of the kettlebell, a good hand insertion does not mean all the weight is in the handle and resting in the palm; there is actually more going on. Part of the weight does indeed rest in the palm downwards, but there is also a part that pulls laterally on the palm and a part that rests on the forearm.

Further explanation follows:
- The majority of weight from the kettlebell should be carried by the palm, wrist, and forearm, not just the forearm (where the bell sits)

With that in mind, it should be noted that due to the design of the kettlebell, it's not possible to completely remove the weight from the forearm

- Practise hand insertion with a kettlebell on the ground or through assisted cleans
- A good hand insert at the corner of the handle (between horn and handle) will change the angle of the bell in relation to your forearm; the round bit of the bell that normally provides the pressure is now positioned differently
- Your fingers do not need to grip around the handle during anything overhead; doing so requires wrist flexion
- Wrist extension might feel like a good thing to do to relieve pressure, but it actually creates more pressure from weight distribution being moved from the forearm to the palm. This might sound good, but too much weight on the palm and hyperextension is also no good
- Condition with light weight; maybe you can press heavier but your forearms are unconditioned to the pressure, so stick with a lighter weight until conditioned
- Tighter grip with the tips of the fingers while all other techniques are perfect might also assist in relieving pressure
- Don't keep pressing with incorrect grip on the kettlebell. Stop, reset, and/or adjust with the other hand
- The more you bring your forearm laterally inwards and away from being vertical, the more pressure will be created
- The more you bring your forearm laterally outward, and away from being vertical, the less pressure on the forearm but more pressure on the shoulder, a position not recommended
- A weak wrist might prompt you to flex it; wrist flexion will increase bell pressure
- If you tried everything, try with a flat open hand (see photo below)

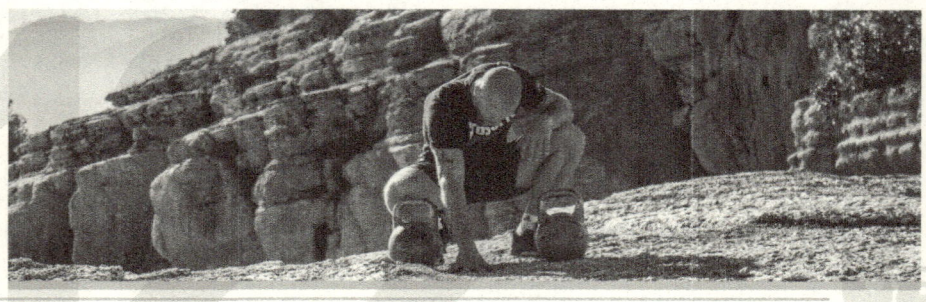

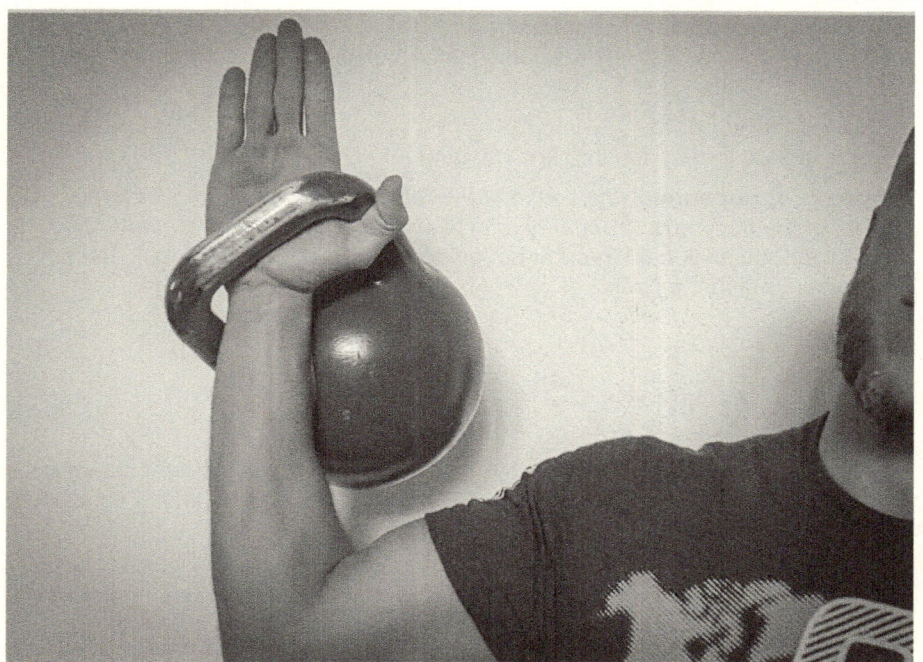

Summary:

- **Transition to hook grip**
  Eliminates calluses

- **Hand rotation/corkscrew**
  Eliminates the kettlebell flipping over the fist, which in turn reduces friction, which reduces calluses

- **Full-arm extension**
  Eliminates constant pressure on the muscles and tendons, which in turn reduces chance of muscle or tendon pain

- **Elbow and body proximity**
  Eliminates banging from the kettlebell coming up too high or landing too far out, which in turn reduces forearm bruising

- **Proper hand insertion**
  Eliminates bending of the wrist, which in turn reduces wrist pain

- **Proper path guidance**
  Eliminates jarring of shoulders, which in turn eliminates one cause for shoulder pain

- **Handle 45 degrees on the back swing**
    Eliminates bobbing of the kettlebell, which prevents friction and reduces calluses

- **Proper and controlled deceleration**
  Eliminates jarring of shoulders, which in turn eliminates one cause for shoulder pain
- **Shortest direct path**
  Helps reduce jarring, friction, and banging
- **Good proprioception** *(the sense of the relative position of neighbouring parts of the body and strength of effort being employed in movement)*
  Helps reduce back pain through not going too low with the kettlebell and not hyper extending the back

SHOULDER PAIN

Shoulder pain can be caused by heavy weights jerking on the shoulders, incorrect lifting, lifting too heavy, uncontrolled quick movements, or performing exercises for which your body is not ready yet.

WRIST PAIN

Wrist pain can be caused by not inserting the hand into the handle properly and having the full weight of the kettlebell rest on the wrist, also referred to as a "broken wrist". Properly inserting the hand into the kettlebell and proper hand rotation will help reduce or eliminate the pain.

KNEE PAIN

Knee pain can be caused by having the feet too close together and pushing the knees outward to allow the kettlebell to travel through the legs, bow legged, or the other way around, the knees buckling in.

ELBOW PAIN

I'm going to generalize things here and refer to it as the elbow area, but there is much more to it. I'm going to cover the elbow joint, brachialis, brachioradialis, and biceps brachii, in particular the tendons which are closely located to the elbow. This whole area is very complex and an area that I see affected the most in beginners.

I'm a firm believer in self-diagnosis, so if you've exhausted the advice of medical professionals and you're still not getting anywhere, I suggest looking into these three muscles – where they're located, when they're worked, and how that relates to your problem.

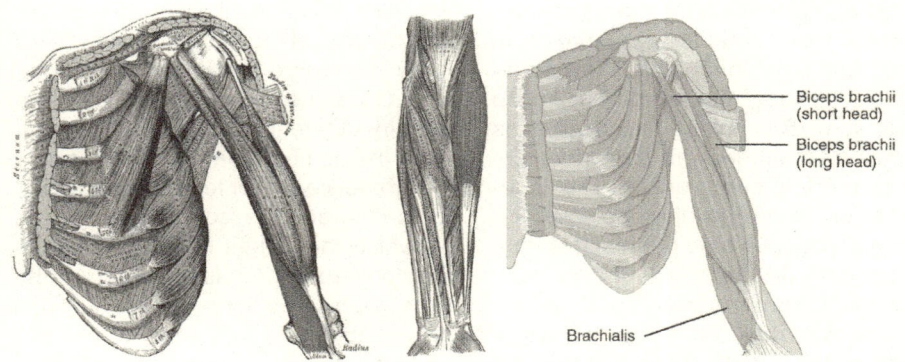

Brachialis, brachioradialis, and biceps brachii.

- All three muscles are responsible for flexing of the arm
- The brachialis is the prime mover of elbow flexion
- The brachioradialis is also capable of pronation and supination of the forearm, which can be seen if you hold your arm out and turn the thumb downwards and back all the way to the right
- The biceps brachii are also capable of supination of the forearm, which you can see in action when you turn your thumb outward

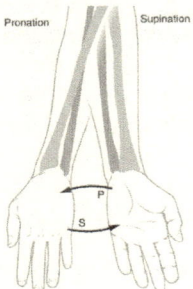

Elbow pain (elbow tendonitis) can be caused by repetitive snapping or jarring of the elbow.

Issues with the tendons of the aforementioned muscles around the elbow area can be caused by a number of things:

- Constant tension on the muscles and tendons due to keeping the elbow bent rather than fully extended on the swing
- Using weights that are too heavy
- Jerking of the arm through uncontrolled descent of the kettlebell
- Casting the kettlebell out rather than a controlled movement
  - Overuse from doing the same thing repeatedly without proper rest
  - Too much too soon when just starting with kettlebells

Appropriate rest is the main prescription for most of these symptoms, but one that most people don't want to do as they feel they're taking a step backward. But unless the problem is rectified, it will go from bad to worse, to completely out of action. This is an extremely annoying injury, so do everything in your power to prevent this from happening; listen to your body, heed the early signs of injury, and reduce any activity that can make the symptoms worse. Finally, work on improving technique and preventing overuse.

Another great prescription is gentle movement without resistance and working on flexibility and range of the muscles affected, thereby preventing them from getting stiff and sore. There are plenty more suggestions like icing, etc. Do some research on your own and try different solutions, but guaranteed the number one remedy is rest.

Another cause for tendon strain could be due to an incorrect racking position in which the weight is constantly pulling forward and causing strain on the elbow flexor tendons. To prevent this from happening, you need to be able to find a proper racking position where the weight is resting on the legs. See the previous section dedicated to racking for more information.

NECK PAIN

Neck pain is usually caused by unnatural positioning of the head during body movement. For example, upon the back swing, you could be staying focused on a point directly in front of you while the rest of your upper body is moving toward the ground, which is putting extreme pressure on your neck. Heavy weights and incorrect body posture, not activating the traps, and no packing of the shoulders and chest could also produce pressure and pain on the neck.

LOWER-BACK PAIN

Make sure you drive the weight up with the legs and hips, not the upper-body, which requires your lower-back to take all the weight. Don't hyper-extend your back on the up part of the swing, but come back up into a neutral standing position.

Make sure you understand what lifting with the back is; understand how not to lift with the back but with the legs, which is through squeezing of the glutes (gluteus maximus) and pressing the heels into the ground. This stance pulls the pelvis up, letting the pelvis lead rather than follow. Your spine should be supported by bracing all core muscles and simply be positioned neutrally upon the pelvis (sacrum, to be exact) and follow along while being powered by the lower body. There is quite a bit more that can be said about this area, which is why I wrote a book about the hip hinge movement which covers exactly this.

KETTLEBELL GOLDEN RULES

Let's go through a few quick and simple rules which, when used consistently, will instantly reduce your chance of injury during kettlebell training:

RULE#1

Never have the kettlebell flip over your fist during the clean. To visualise, imagine the kettlebell resting on your forearm, with your fist pointed up to the ceiling (racking position). Now imagine the kettlebell flipping onto the other side of your fist (i.e.,

on the inside of your forearm or vice versa). The kettlebell flipping over the fist is what I see regularly with beginners who try to perform the clean, or when they cast the kettlebell out from racking position.

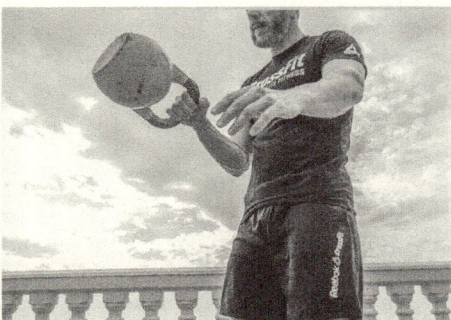 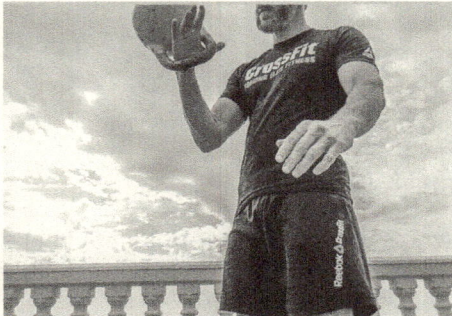

RULE#2

Never hold the handle too tight. Doing so can cause muscle pain or cramps in your forearm. Hold the kettlebell loosely but with just enough force to stay in control at all times. Grabbing the handle too tightly when doing snatches will also drastically increase your chances of ripping your calluses – when your calluses are ripped, you are likely out of commission for at least a week or two.

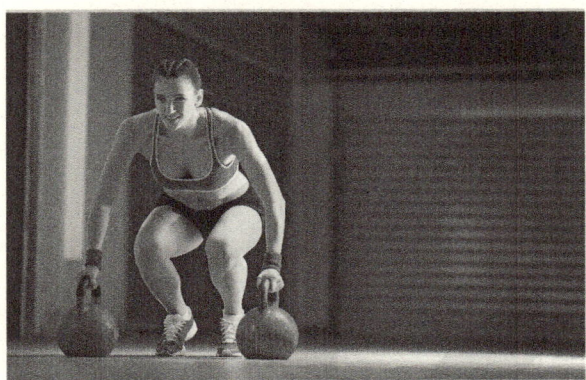

RULE#3

Never rest the kettlebell weight on your palm. Meaning, an incorrect hand insert which puts all the weight on the wrist. The kettlebell should also rest on your forearm, or forearm and bicep, depending to what exercise you're transitioning. These positions will distribute the weight to the ball of your hand, forearm, and bicep.

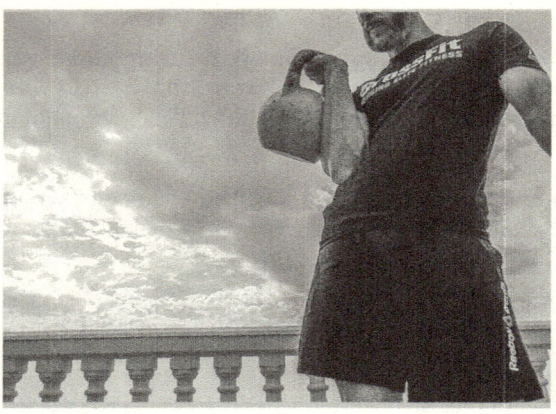

RULE#4

Always use your lower body to clean the kettlebell. If you're using your upper body by bicep curling your kettlebell up, you run the risk of muscle or tendon injuries. Not fully extending the arm on the swing, and keeping the muscles under constant tension can also produce muscle and tendon problems. Note that tendonitis can also be caused by over-use.

RULE#5

Never position the hand on the outside of the elbow in racking position. The elbow should be positioned close to the ribs with the hand on or near the middle of the chest.

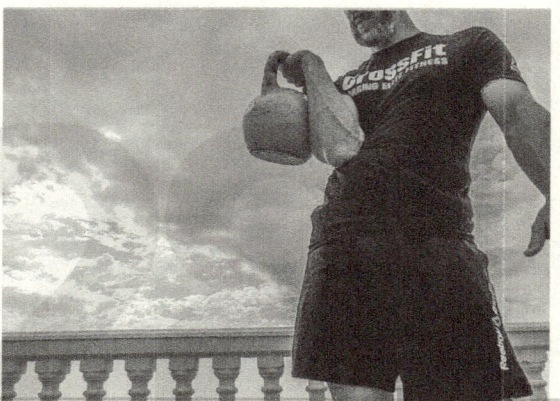

RULE#6

Communication is of the utmost importance. Communicate with your trainer or from whomever you receive guidance. If something does not feel right, hurts, or is uncomfortable, the trainer cannot always see this. Express your issues, never feel shy or afraid to ask questions, and remember, there are no stupid questions.

RULE#7

Never try and rescue a bad repetition. You will only risk injuring yourself. If the rep is bad and out of control, drop it safely or bring it down to ground in as controlled a manner as possible. The kettlebell does not break, and the gym where you work out should care more about your safety than their equipment.

RULE#8

Preferably wear no shoes at all during kettlebell training. If you must wear shoes because of gym rules (get a new gym), choose flat shoes. I do not recommend wearing running shoes; you will risk ankle and knee injuries. Bare feet will not only improve your kettlebell training but will also improve your balance, your ankle and foot strength, plus your toes will love you for it.

RULE#9

Learn to perfect the hip hinge dead lift. Then move on to the kettlebell swing and once the swing is perfected, move on to the clean. Each exercise builds upon the previous one, so follow the path.

RULE#10

Never do renegade rows on classic kettlebells. Use competition kettlebells for this exercise, unless you're in an advanced state and looking for that extra added stability. Classic kettlebells have a small surface base which makes it very easy for them to topple over and injure your wrists, while the competition kettlebells have a big enough base to make the kettlebell stable enough to support your body weight.

OVERHEAD PRESS

The kettlebell press is another exercise you'll be wanting to master when you get started with kettlebell training. I've written a whole book about the subject with Joe Daniels that is well worth reading if you want to learn the finer details on pressing. I'm going to cover the most common reason for injury with the overhead press in this book for you.

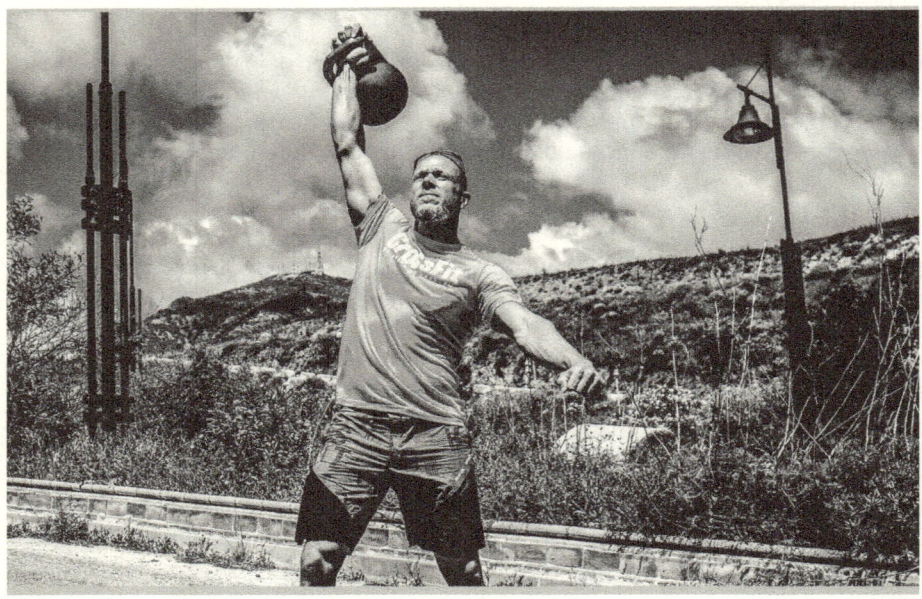

The three main areas affected with shoulder pressing are the rotator cuff and front and side delts, the most common causes being:

- Pressing too heavy
- Pressing with incorrect hand insert
- Pressing through an inefficient path
- Pressing too much

Pressing too heavy is one that has to do primarily with ego. For some reason, anyone that steps into the gym wants to pick up the heaviest kettlebell and press it overhead, even if it means turning red in the face, arching the back, and injuring the shoulder. Don't get caught up into this; progress safely and stay in the game.

I've covered a good hand insert extensively, but it's just as important with pressing. Don't get complacent with an incorrect hand insert just because you're pressing 8kg, 10kg, or other light weight. Even if the insert seems not to affect you, it will with overuse and/or when going up in weight, and it might even hold you back from progressing to pressing heavier weight.

When you first start pressing, you should become familiar with the best and most efficient path to take from racking to end position overhead. This is the path you want to adhere to while training, and from there progress to different angles with more weight. An efficient and direct path does not put unconditioned muscles under dangerous or damaging strain.

Efficient and safest pressing path:
- ✔ Direct straight line from rack to overhead
- ✔ Looking side-on the bell does not travel outwards
  the kettlebell does not travel away from the body, other than upwards
- ✔ Looking front-on the bell does not travel laterally

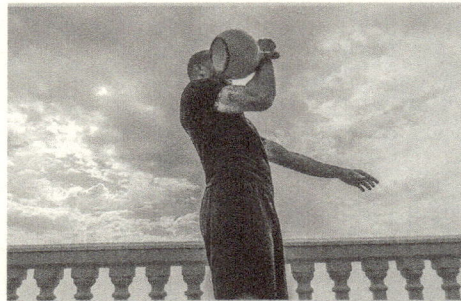
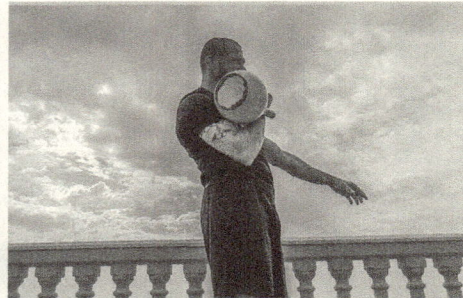

Good racking position. Press.

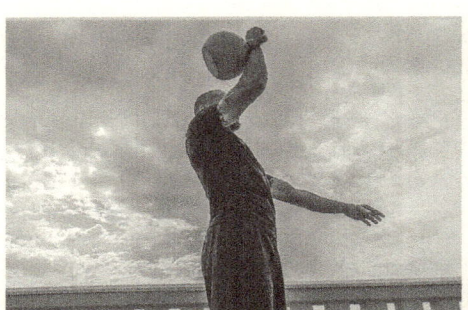
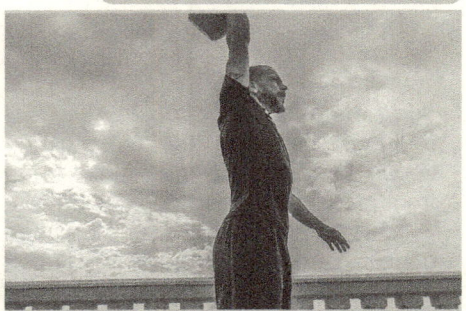

Direct path to overhead. Full lockout.

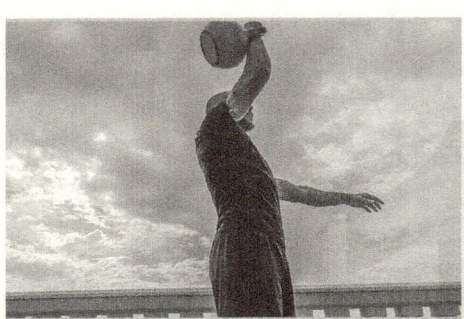
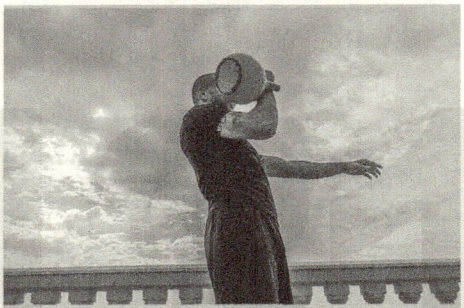

Bring the bell down. Make space.

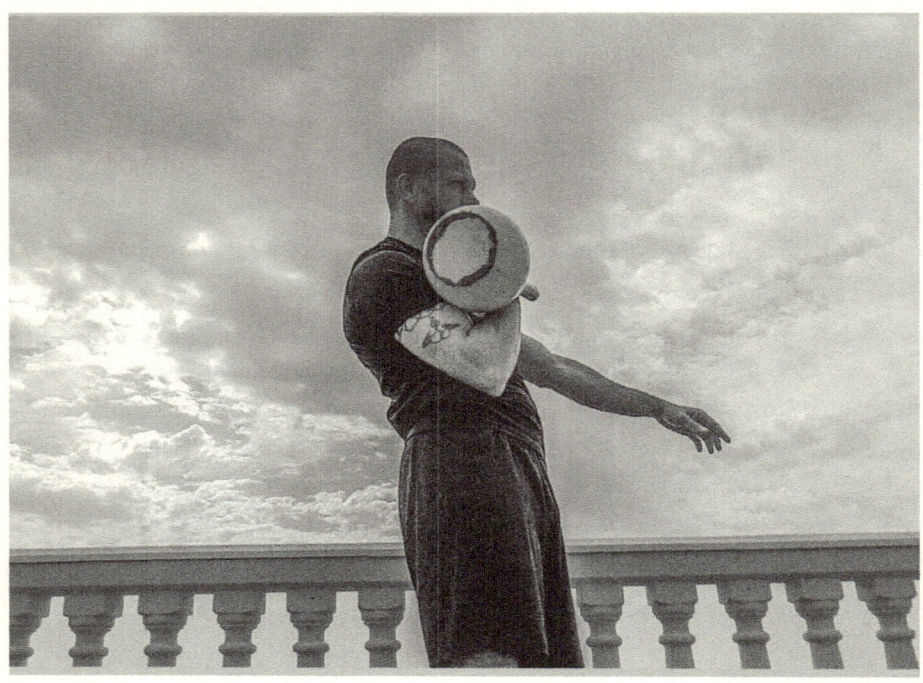

Rack and repeat.

For the majority of people, the front (anterior) delts are the most conditioned for pressing, thus making the front press the safest progression with which to start. In everyday life, when people need to put objects high upon a shelf, they will take the direct path up; they're not going to press out to the side (working the side delt) to put the object in place. Therefore, when starting to overhead press, learn the front press first, then progress to the hybrid and then side press.

When progressing to different angles, don't use the same weight you're already pressing, in other words, if you're easily pressing 16kg in the front press, don't use the same weight for the side press; start with 10 or 12kg.

A good overhead lockout is important for a good press, meaning the weight rests on the skeletal system in lockout, rather than on the muscular system. A bent arm means the weight is resting on the muscles; a locked out arm means the weight can also rest on the skeletal system. A good lockout requires overhead flexibility and mobility. This is what you should work on with light weight before progressing in weight.

KETTLEBELL ROWS

The kettlebell row might feel a little out of place in this book, but I want to cover it, as kettlebell back exercises are usually overlooked. It seems more like a thing to do in bodybuilding. I'm of the opposite opinion, however, and include a lot of rowing work with my clients and classes. That said, I like to cover the most common mistakes made with most rowing exercises, whether with a kettlebell or barbell.

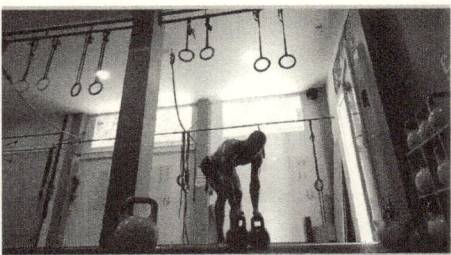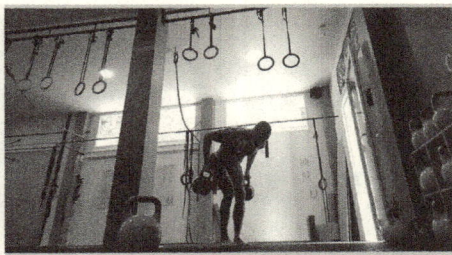

Bent-over dead rows

There is a reoccurring mistake I see people make when doing kettlebell bent-over rows, and it means that they're not working the muscles they intended to work.

Rows are a pulling exercise and are supposed to work the back, and with kettlebells you also 100% involve the core and legs with each variation. Unlike machines, there is nothing to hold you up, lean against, or sit on, thus you need to hold yourself up.

The odd thing about this exercise is that the range feels very short; this is just a feeling; however, it will cause a lot of people to pull the kettlebell up too far — don't over-exaggerate the range by pulling it up too far. Your elbows should come just past your ribs and that's enough. If you're a coach, you'll want to provide a cue for your clients at which point to stop.

Let's talk about the number one mistake most people make when performing the kettlebell row. If you want to see it done intentionally, watch my video here: youtube.com/watch?v=W-pK-4gjaKoI&t=5m9s, another example is in this video: youtube.com/watch?v=tiC0zyITB0w&t=3m15s. Kettlebell rows are designed to target the back, the rear delts, and rhomboids. The main mistake is that some people work their biceps rather than the target muscles, but this is not a problem if you were planning to work your biceps!

The proper way to row is to relax the forearm and have it do nothing more than hold the weight. You do not want to feel your biceps, or anything in the anterior compartment of the upper-arm for that matter; you want to focus on the rear delts or other back muscles, depending on what variation of the row you're performing.

KETTLEBELL ROW VARIATIONS

- **Renegade rows**
  Double-arm, dead

- **Bent-over rows wide (90°)**
  Single-arm or double-arm, dead or hang

- **Bent-over rows hybrid (45°)**
  Single-arm or double-arm, dead or hang

- **Bent-over rows narrow (0°)**
  Single-arm or double-arm, dead or hang

For the bent-over rows you can hip hinge with bent knees or locked-out knees. The degrees refer to the angle between the elbow and ribs.

- **Squat rows**
  Single-arm or double-arm, dead or hang

- **Long lunge rows**
  Single-arm, dead or hang

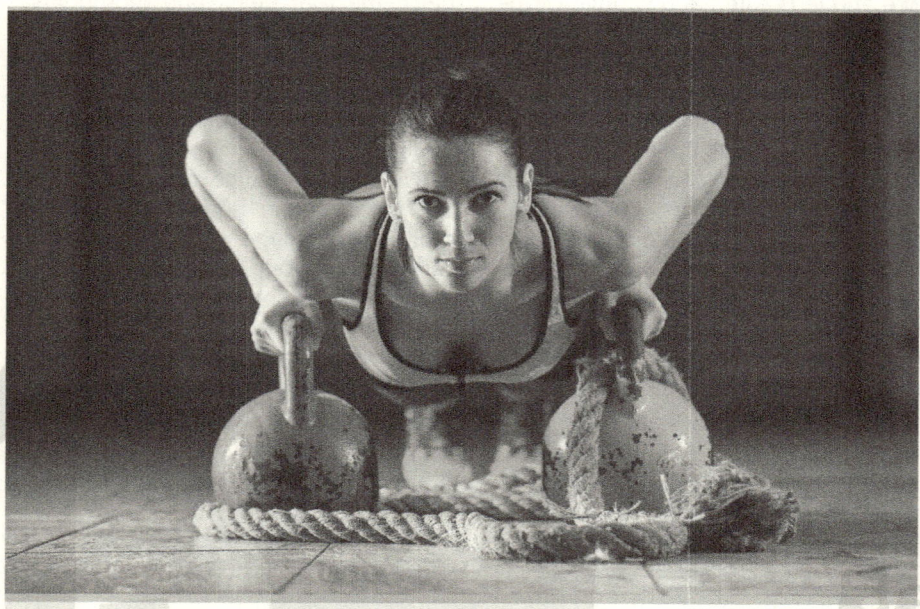

MUSCLES WORKED WITH ROWS

- Rhomboids
- Rear deltoids
- Triceps
- Erector spinae
- Trapezius
- Other core muscles

Now you know you can also work your biceps with rows when you do them incorrectly, or if you intentionally want to work them with rows, that's all right as well.

- **Wide** works more the rhomboids and rear delts
- **Narrow** works more the tricep and rear delts
- **Renegade** rows works more the triceps, rear delts, lats, and core
- **Long** lunge rows works more the triceps, rear delts, and quads
- **Squat** rows works more the triceps, rear delts, and quads
- **Dead** rows are longer range but relieve tension on the muscles for a short period
- **Hang** rows are shorter range but keep tension on the muscles

You can perform a long lunge row while resting the forearm arm on the knee, or resting the extended arm on the kettlebell. The latter provides greater stability.

The bent-over row single kettlebell double-arm is the easiest version of all rows.

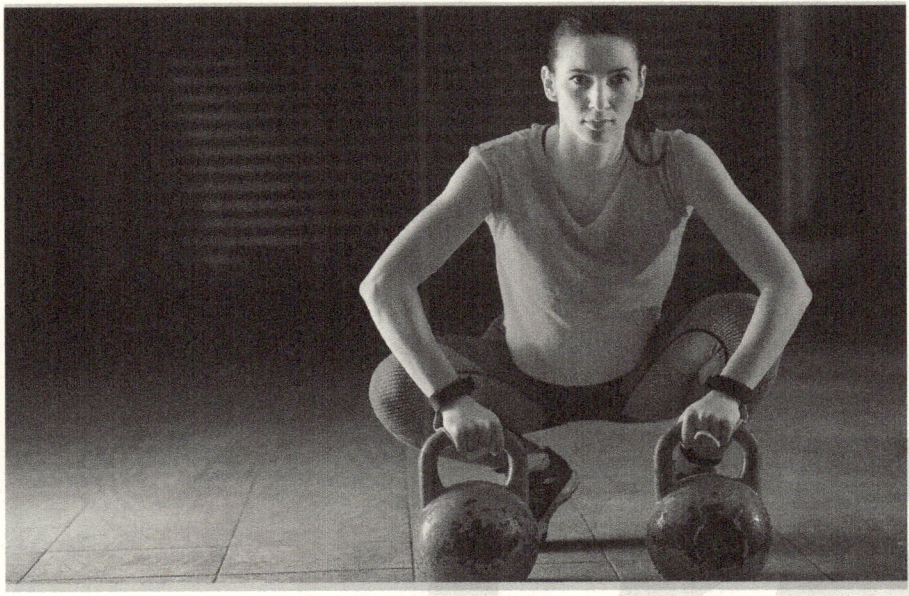

STRETCHING

The difference between static and dynamic stretching is that you stretch the muscle and immediately shorten it in a dynamic stretch. Examples of dynamic stretches are hip hinges, lunges, and squats. Examples of static stretches are coming into a lunge and holding it, coming into a squat and holding it, etc.

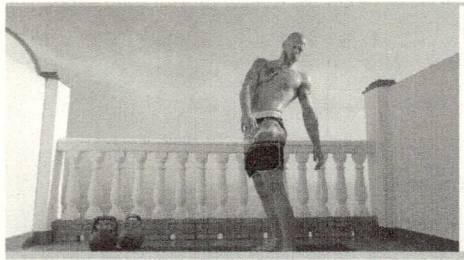
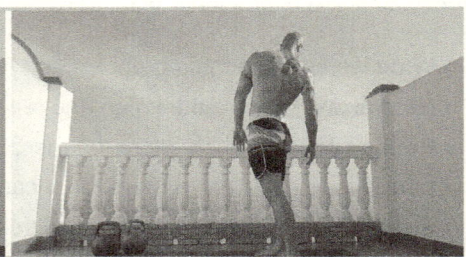

Stretching is just as important as the warm-up and exercise itself; with better flexibility comes better performance and less chance of injury. After each workout, you should take some time to stretch; in fact, the longer you can devote to stretching, the better your body will perform for you.

Following are the areas you want to pay particular attention to when stretching:

- Hip flexors
- Hamstrings
- Quadriceps
- Forearms / biceps
- Pectoralis
- Deltoids
- Triceps
- Latissimus dorsi
- Gluteus maximus
- Adductors and abductors

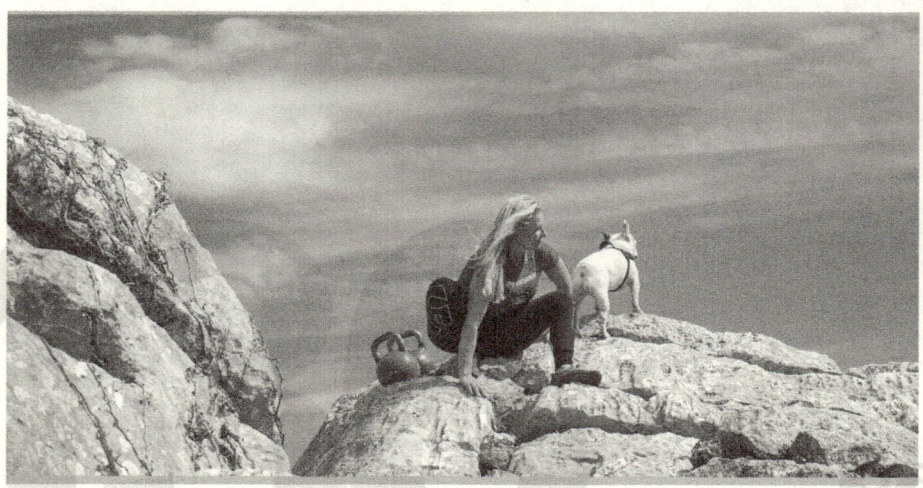

Following are some basic stretches recommended to include in your stretching regime after your workouts:

- **Butterfly Stretch**
  Adductors
- **Lizard Pose**
  Hamstrings, quads, adductors and hip flexors
- **Tipover Tuck Hamstring Stretch**
  Hamstrings and front deltoids
- **Easy Quad Stretch / Lying Side Quad Stretch**
  Quadriceps
- **Kneeling Forearm / Bicep Stretch**
  Forearms and biceps
- **Single Arm Chest Stretch**
  Pectoralis and front deltoids
- **Posterior Shoulder Stretch**
  Rear deltoids
- **Overhead Tricep Stretch**
  Triceps
- **Overhead Lat Stretch**
  Triceps and latissimus dorsi
- **Seated Leg Hug**
  Gluteus maximus

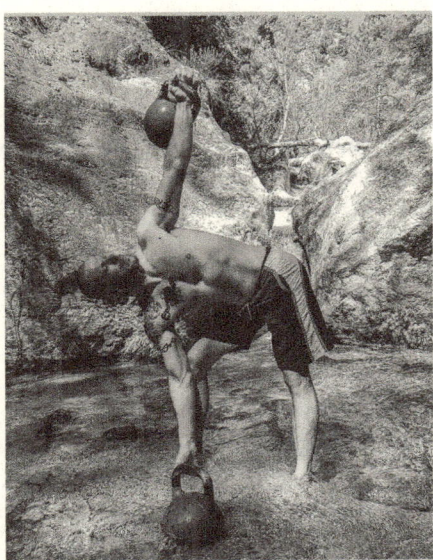

Double kettlebell windmi

BUTTERFLY STRETCH

Main target(s): adductors

Seated on the ground, bring your heels together and pull them toward your body by grabbing your shins at the bottom (just above the foot), place your elbows on the inside thighs and gently push the knees towards the ground while keeping the chest out and back straight.

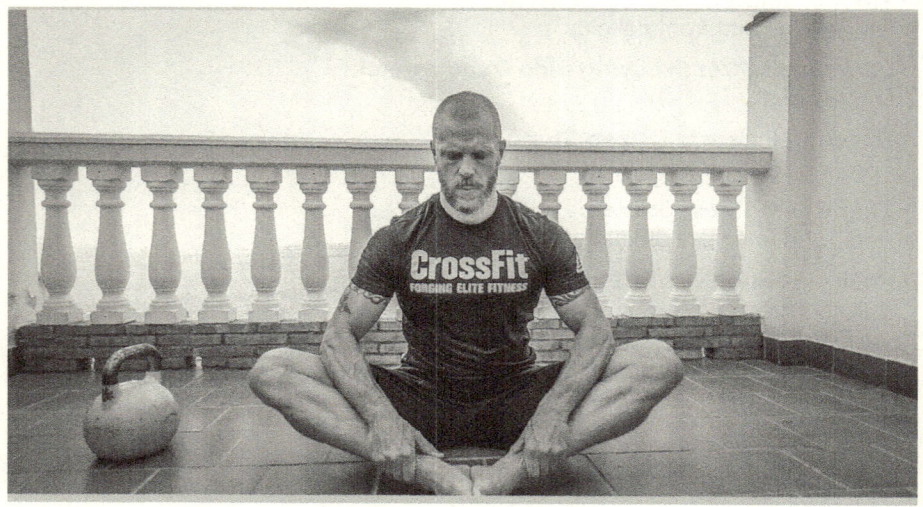

LIZARD POSE

Main target(s): hamstrings, quads, adductors, and hip flexors

Start in a plank position with your hands placed right under your shoulders, elbows locked out. Bring the right foot forward, and place it close to the right hand or past if flexibility allows. Keep the spine in a neutral position, push the hips slightly down, squeeze the glutes, and push the back foot into the ground. Repeat on the other side.

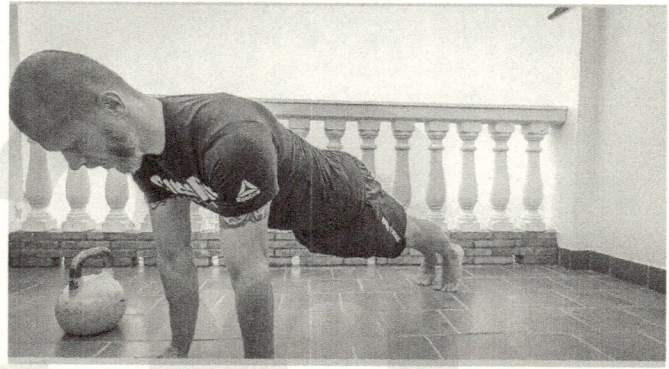

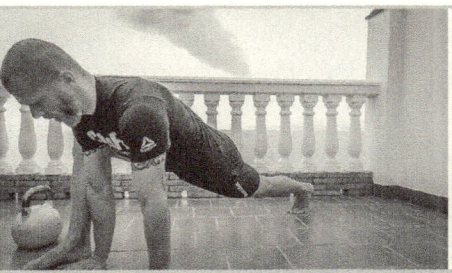 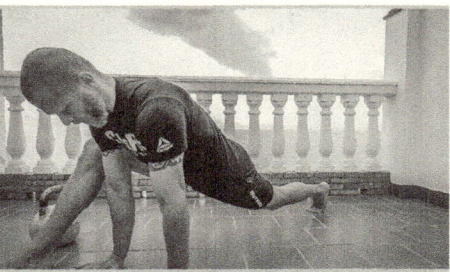

Lizard pose. Deeper stretch.

TIPOVER TUCK HAMSTRING STRETCH

Main target(s): hamstrings and front deltoids

Stand straight with the feet in neutral position, finger interlocked behind the body. Slowly lower the torso toward the ground, bending at the hips, leaving the knees locked out. Come to the lowest position possible without putting pressure on the spine, and bring the hands towards the head.

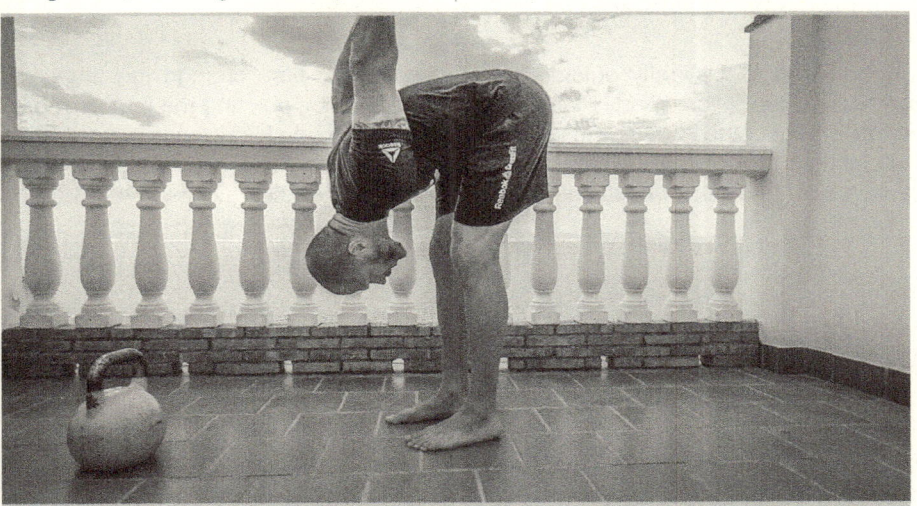

EASY QUAD STRETCH / LYING SIDE QUAD STRETCH

Main target(s): quadriceps

This stretch can be performed standing up or lying down on your side. Stand straight with the feet in neutral position. Bring one foot toward the buttocks; grab with one hand the bottom of the shin just above the foot. Keep the knee active, not loose. Pull the heel into the buttocks and push the hip forward. Repeat on the other side.

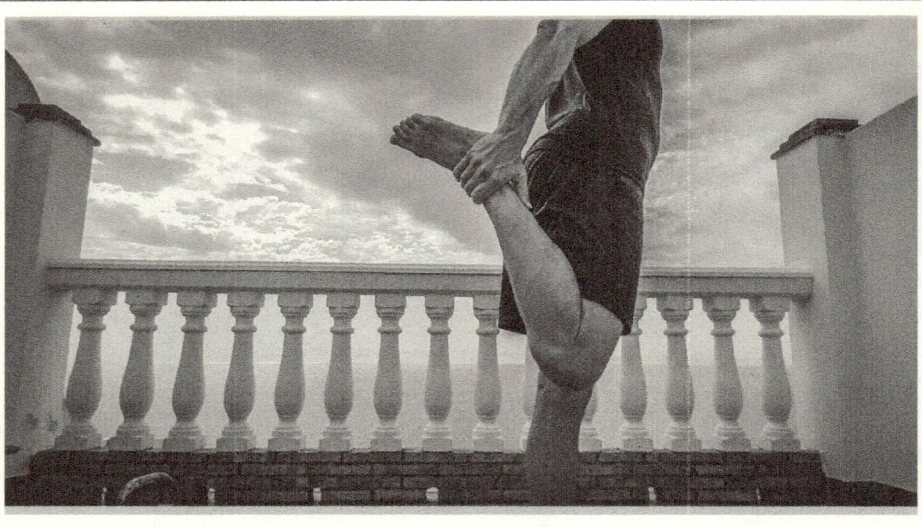

KNEELING FOREARM / BICEP STRETCH

Main target(s): forearms and biceps

Kneel, with feet slightly outside the buttocks, knees wide apart. Place the hands in front of the knees, with the fingers pointing toward your body. Gently sit back; push the chest out. After a period of time change the angle of the hands by pointing the fingers more inward (i.e., pinkies closer to each other).

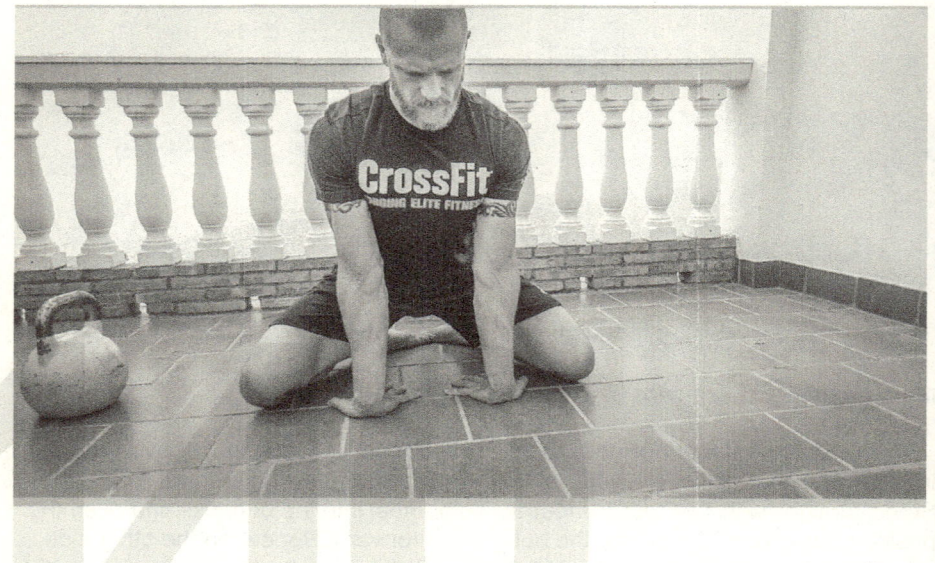

SINGLE ARM CHEST STRETCH

Main target(s): pectoralis and front deltoids

Stand in front of a wall. Place one hand flat on the wall in line with your shoulder. You want the fingers pointing out towards the side. Now start turning away from the wall with your torso by moving your feet first. Look away from the wall. Keep turning as far as possible while keeping the hand connected to the wall, and try to bring the opposite shoulder towards the pinkie of the hand on the wall.

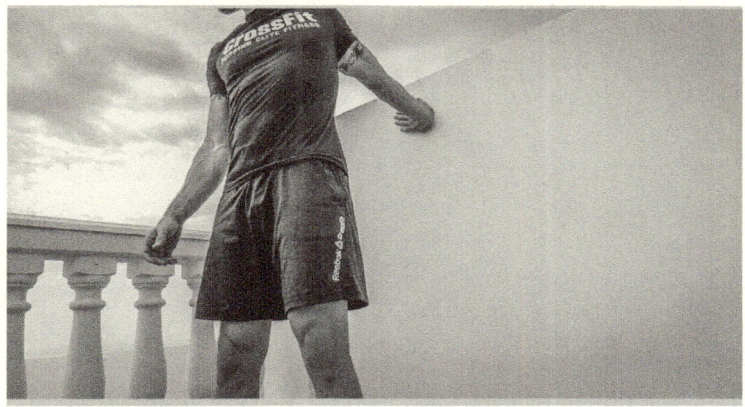

POSTERIOR SHOULDER STRETCH

Main target(s): rear deltoids

Stand straight with the feet in neutral position. Pull the right lat down to pull the shoulder away from the ear, which assists in achieving a more effective stretch. Bring the right arm across the body, in line with the shoulder. Hug that arm with the left arm around the elbow area of the right arm, and gently pull the right arm toward the left shoulder. Repeat on the other side.

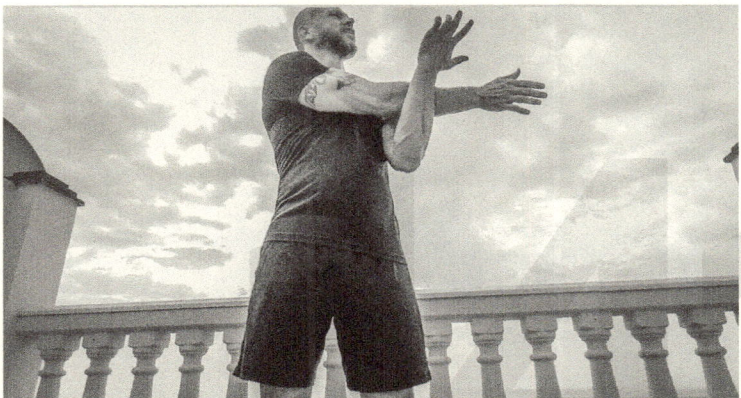

OVERHEAD TRICEP STRETCH

Main target(s): triceps

Stand straight with the feet in neutral position. Bring the right arm straight up into the air, bend the elbow, and bring the right hand behind your head. Grab the right elbow with the left hand, and gently pull the elbow toward the left shoulder while moving the right hand down across the spine. Repeat on the other side.

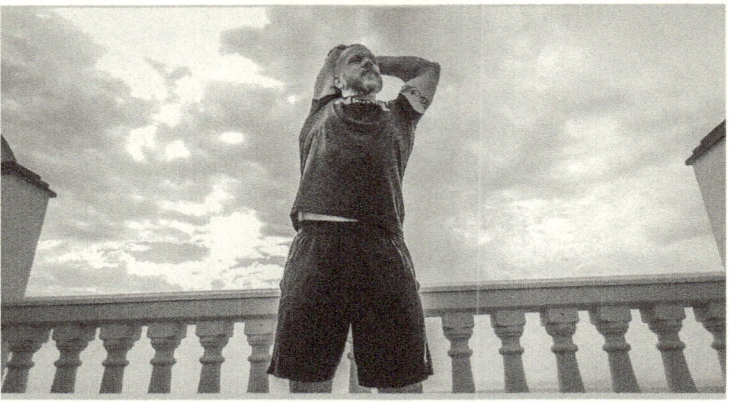

OVERHEAD LAT STRETCH

Main target(s): triceps and latissimus dorsi

Perform the same stretch as the tricep stretch, but this time put the feet a little wider apart and gently push the hips to one side, and bend into the stretch while maintaining a super tight core. Perform this stretch slowly and controlled. Repeat on the other side.

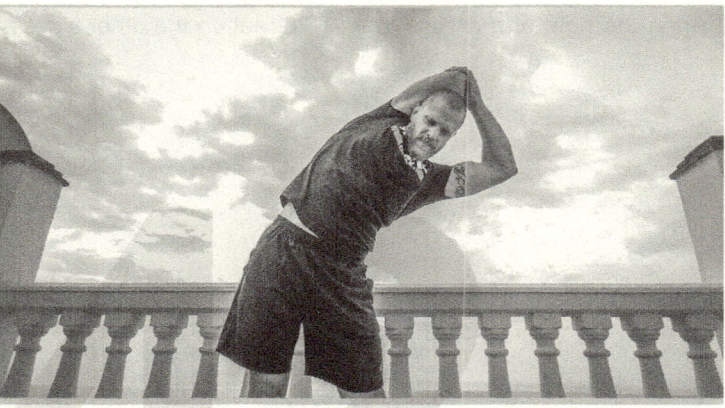

SEATED LEG HUG

Main target(s): gluteus maximus

Sit down on the floor with the legs straight out. Move the right foot over the left leg; place it as close as possible to the left hip. Hug the right leg with the left arm just under the knee area. Gently pull the right knee toward the left shoulder while pressing the buttocks into the floor. Repeat on the other side.

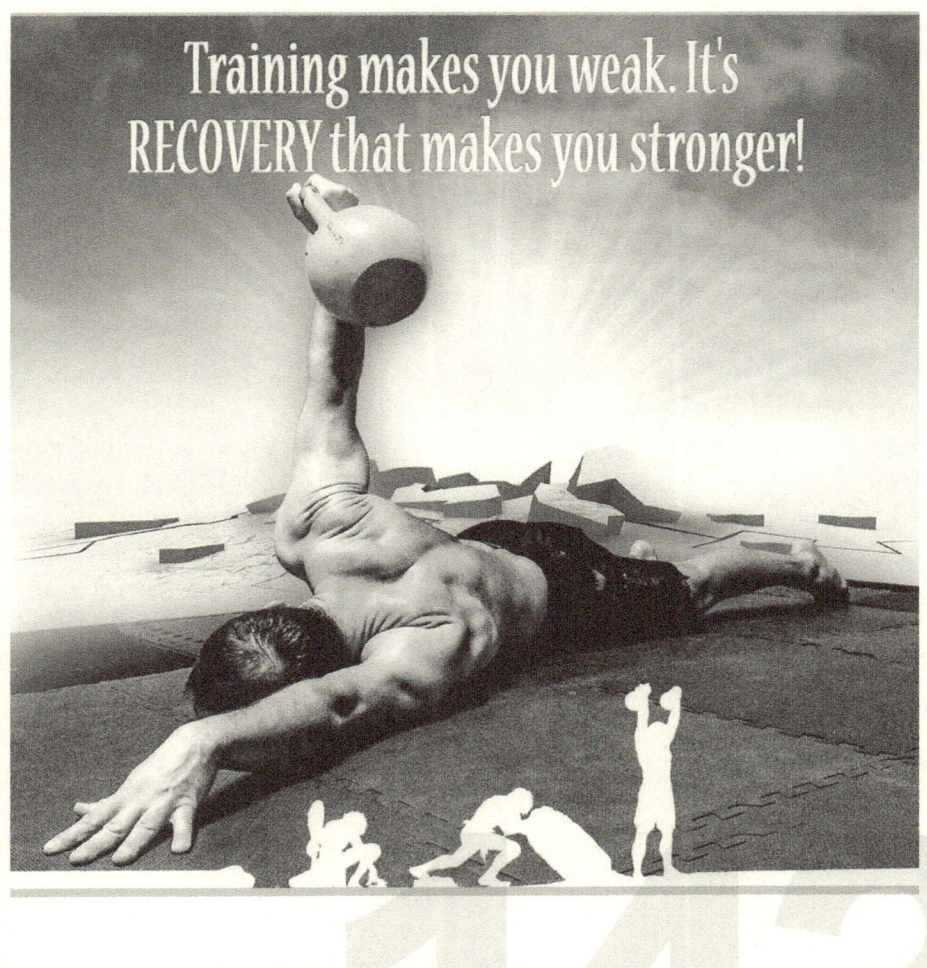

BECOME CERTIFIED

As the owner of Cavemantraining I would like to congratulate you on having finished reading one of the most detailed kettlebell training books for laying the proper foundations. Why not take the next step to becoming a PRO kettlebell enthusiast or trainer? Complete and receive your certificate for one of the most detailed kettlebell courses available, I'd be extremely proud to be part of your progression.

Take the online course and become a certified kettlebell trainer:

WWW.CAVEMANTRAINING.COM/LEARN-KETTLEBELLS-HOME/

BIG THANKS

Big thanks to those who took the time to provide an early review on the book.

Ken Edds – Baton Rouge, Louisiana USA

Mark Godwin, Director Fit biz UK

Bryan Trish

Don Brown

PROOFREADING

David Van Der Molen

OPPORTUNITY

Want to translate this book into another language?

Contact me at me@tacofleur.com and let's discuss revenue share.

OVERSEAS KETTLEBELL ADVENTURES

I'm from the Netherlands, Amsterdam, but I've lived in Spain, Australia, Vietnam, Thailand, and now back in Spain permanently. I'm available to run workshops and also outdoor kettlebell fitness adventures, whether solo; family; group; or team building, hikes, boot camps, and challenges. www.youtube.com/watch?v=BsTyeZOKM5c

Contact me to discuss at me@tacofleur.com or via Facebook at www.facebook.com/taco.fleur.

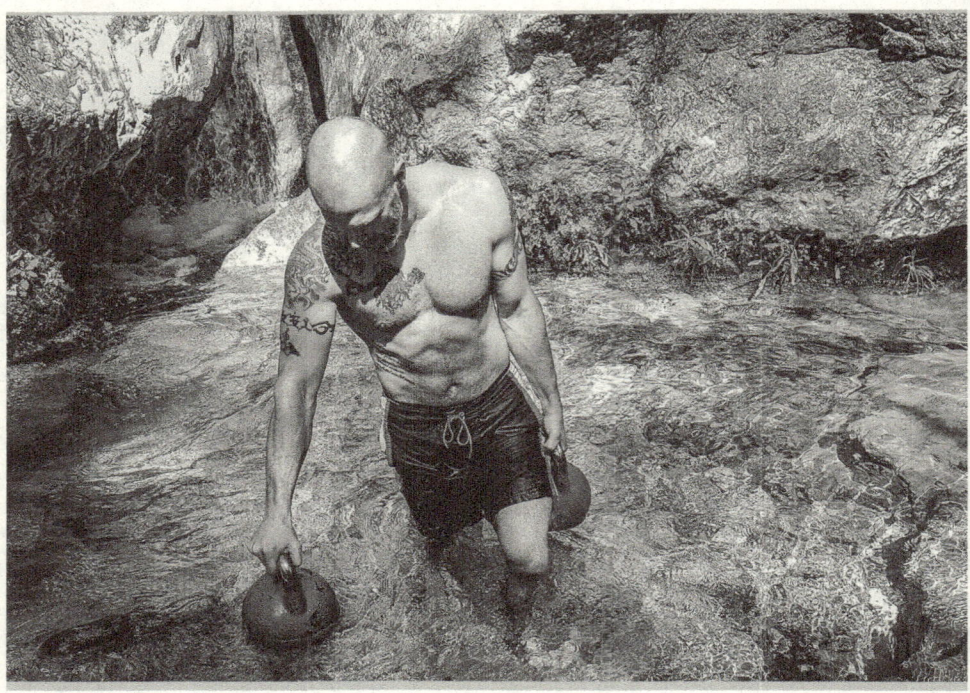

PARTNERS AND SPONSORS.

www.facebook.com/caveman.kettlebells

www.cavemantraining.com

www.facebook.com/groups/kettlebell.enthusiasts/

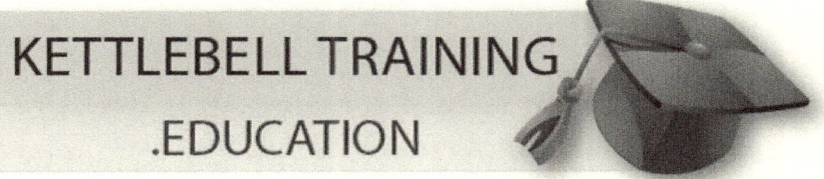

kettlebelltraining.education

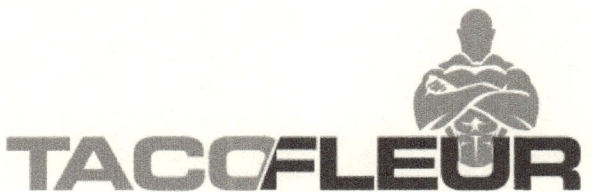

www.tacofleur.com

Made in the USA
Coppell, TX
30 November 2020

42443995R10090